SI KING AND DAVE MYERS

THE HAIRY *Dieters*

SIMPLE HEALTHY FOOD

CONT

SIMPLE
HEALTHY
FOOD

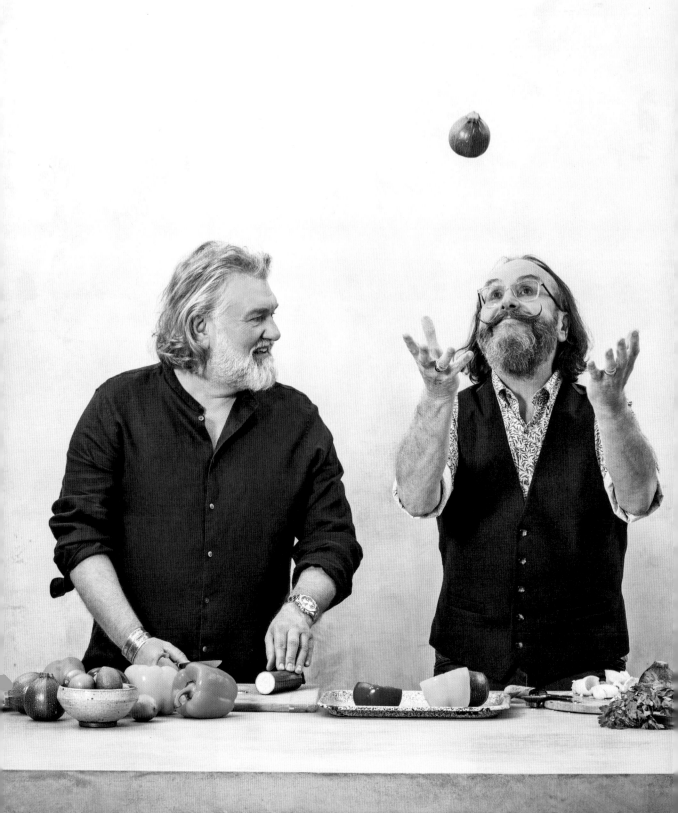

ENTS

TEN YEARS ON – WHAT'S RIGHT AND WHAT'S NOT?

It's ten years since we made our 'Hairy Dieters' television series and published our first 'Hairy Dieters' book – a time that changed our lives. Before then we were, to put it bluntly, obese. While we will never be super-skinny, we've kept to a better weight and improved our blood sugar levels and cholesterol. We've changed our cooking style to include more veg and lighter dishes and we're definitely way healthier than we were back then.

We've stopped sticking our heads in the sand and we're well aware of the risks of carrying too much timber. It's not about looking like you're auditioning for 'Love Island' – it's to do with good health. Being overweight or obese increases the risk of many illnesses, including type 2 diabetes, high blood pressure, heart disease and strokes, as well as cancer. And the older you get, the more important it is to stay at a healthy weight. Research has shown links between excess weight and ten types of cancer, including bowel, kidney and cervical, and it's thought that weight problems are behind about 18,000 cases of cancer a year in the UK. It's that serious.

But, as you all know, we love cooking and we love our food and that's never going to change. In our 'Hairy Dieters' books, we've focused on showing that you can stay healthy and maintain a good weight while still enjoying proper tasty meals and having fun with your cooking. The secret is to eat well but not too much – watch your portion size and keep the amount of fat, sugar and carbs to sensible levels.

A lot has happened in ten years, and we realise that new research has meant that some dietary advice has changed and moved on. We try our best to keep up, but it's easy to get confused by the endless bombardment of info – don't eat carbs, eat carbs, go high-fibre, low fat, and so on. Every week there seems to be new advice about diet and health – often very contradictory – and it can be hard to know what's right and what isn't. It would be all too easy just to give up and reach for the nearest biscuit, but that's not the answer.

Before we wrote the recipes for this book, we wanted some straightforward, up-to-date info to cut through all the confusion, so we got in touch with our old friend Professor Roy Taylor. He worked with us when we started on this journey and he's one of the most reliable experts on all things to do with diet through his work on type 2 diabetes. He set us straight on the questions that were puzzling us – and maybe you too. What he told us helped us get the right balance of health and deliciousness in our recipes.

Dave: Ten years ago, the mantra was cut the calories, move more and you'll lose weight, but I know that some people now say that counting calories is not the way to do it. I find it helpful though, and I think many people do, so is it still a valid way to manage your weight?

Prof Roy: It's certainly important to be aware of calories. Look at the labels and when you see that some tempting snack is actually 400 calories maybe you will put it back! People need a practical way of organising what they eat. Some foods are very high in calories and recognising this is crucial. Often, they are things that slip down easily yet still leave you hungry after a couple of hours: the danger foods. But counting calories every time you eat is just too much for most of us.

Once you know which are the danger foods, simply avoiding these and watching how much you eat can be enough to avoid weight gain. And if you stick to a good mix of vegetables and fruit as well as protein foods, you will find it easier to reduce the number of calories you consume. In particular, processed foods and ready meals contain lots of salt and sugar to encourage you to eat more of them – and buy them again and again. The sugar in these foods is invisible and so just loads you with added calories with no benefit to your health or effect on your appetite. In studies in which people are left to choose what they want to eat from a selection of fresh foods or of processed foods, the group eating processed foods consumed more calories. Processed food is also lower in fibre and it's important to get plenty of fibre in our diet.

Dave: Remind me why fibre is so important.

Prof Roy: Fibre is good for the gut and helps us feel full and satisfied. There's fibre in fruit and vegetables and eating plenty of these foods is important. Fibre in bran and wholemeal breads is also a Good Thing. Fibre-rich food provides bulk, which helps your bowels work properly. Processed food and ready meals typically do not contain fibre, so they are less satisfying and not good for your system.

Si: In our earlier *Hairy Dieters* books we always recommended low-fat yoghurt, cheese and so on. Is that still the thing to do or has the advice changed?

Prof Roy: Opinions have moved on here and most experts now agree that you don't need to go for low-fat foods, many of which contain added sugar. But – and it is a big but – fat is high in calories, and it's all too easy to eat too much of it. The Mediterranean diet is the one most often shown to be beneficial – plenty of vegetables and wholegrains, plus small amounts of meat, dairy and olive oil – and research shows that it is a diet most people can stick to quite easily. If you want some cheese or yoghurt, go for the full-fat stuff which has better flavour, is a more natural food and less processed. But enjoy it in moderation.

Dave: I've always been told that breakfast is the most important meal of the day. Is that true?

Prof Roy: It depends on your metabolism. Some people find it impossible to function without eating breakfast. Others are fine with just a cup of coffee. There's no metabolic reason why anyone must eat at a certain time of day, so go with what feels right for you. If you do eat breakfast, include some protein. A heavy carb load is the very worst way to start the day.

Si: And what about carbohydrates? Is a low-carb diet the way to go?

Prof Roy: What many people don't realise is that excess carbs turn to sugar in the body. The excess is stored in the liver where it becomes 100 per cent saturated fat. But I'm certainly not saying avoid carbs totally. Some of us do well on a low-carb diet but not all. Instead, aim for a carb intake of less than 40 per cent of your total diet – that still allows you to have a bit of cake for tea. In the UK, we tend to average about 45 per cent, whereas in most other European countries it's more like 40 per cent. You need some carbs to keep the system ticking over and it's good to have carbs with a bit of roughage, like brown rice and wholemeal bread, but even with these your digestion turns them into sugar. It doesn't matter whether they are brown or white. In today's world, moderately reducing the amount of carbs you eat is wise.

Dave: So what's the story on fruit? I know it can raise your blood sugar but it's also good for you, isn't it?

Prof Roy: Fruit is great, but fruit juice is not. It's stuffed with calories and no fibre. Just think about it: you might drink the juice of eight oranges in one go, but you would be very unlikely to eat eight whole oranges in one sitting. Whole fresh fruit, though, is a great food and although it contains sugar, it is a slow-release carb and contains lots of nutrients. Keep it unprocessed and go easy if you are at risk of diabetes.

Si: We both eat lots of veggie food now, but we do enjoy a bit of meat and fish as well. Is that OK?

Prof Roy: Absolutely. Meat and fish are fantastic foods and it's fine to have some as part of a healthy diet. If you can, go for some good-quality meat and sustainable fish, but aim to have some veggie days every week.

Si: What about the 'five-a-day' mantra? Some people think it's OK to do this by having lots of fruit and smoothies, but I guess that's not a good idea?

Prof Roy: It is not. There's no point in stuffing yourself with fruit juice and smoothies while carrying on eating cake and stodge. I prefer to suggest 'five insteads a day'. So *instead* of a slice of apple pie you have an apple; *instead* of a side of chips you have some delicious leeks or a serving of pulses. That's a definite win-win, as the result is that you have more of the good stuff and less of the bad.

Dave: I've done crash diets in the past, but is it better to lose weight gradually? And is it true that your metabolism slows down if you do a crash diet?

Prof Roy: Studies show that it is better for people to diet for a defined period – perhaps for about two months to lose a good amount of weight. Then once you've reached your goal, start on a weight-maintenance diet to prevent regain. People generally find this easier to cope with – you don't want to feel you're going to be dieting forever, just for a limited time. It's nice to know there is an end in sight and severely restricting calories gets you to your goal quicker, so is encouraging.

And your metabolism doesn't slow down but after dieting, you are smaller, so you need fewer calories to maintain your new weight. A reasonable aim for a weight-loss phase would be about 800 calories a day.

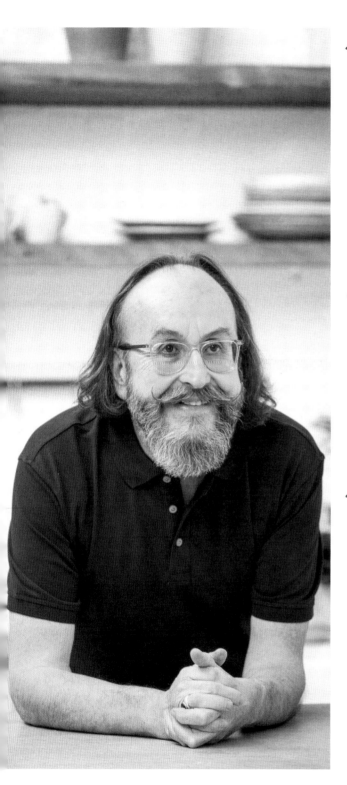

Dave: OK, so once you're at a healthy weight, what sort of calorie count should you aim for to maintain weight?

Prof Roy: On average, it would be about 2,000 calories for a woman and 2,500 for a man. But there is a huge variation in this, and it depends very much on your body size and amount of physical activity. You'll soon know if you're eating too much and putting the weight back on. It's a good idea not to overdo your evening meal. Aim to keep it under 700–1,000 calories.

Si: And what about alcohol? Can we enjoy the odd drink?

Prof Roy: Yes. Life is for living. But if alcohol intake becomes too regular, then It's trouble. The problem is that often people don't realise the calorie count of alcoholic drinks. It's high and those excess calories are stored as fat in the body. I advise no alcohol during a weight-loss phase and then enjoy it in moderation once you're at your target weight.

Dave: And how much water should we drink?

Prof Roy: Drink when you're thirsty, but don't feel you have to drink large amounts. Your body has a great system for telling you if it needs extra fluids. It is, though, a very good idea to have a glass of water when you feel hungry. The water fills you up and the moment passes – without piling in extra calories.

Prof Roy: Now it's my turn to ask the questions! What do you both find is the hardest thing about staying healthy and watching your weight?

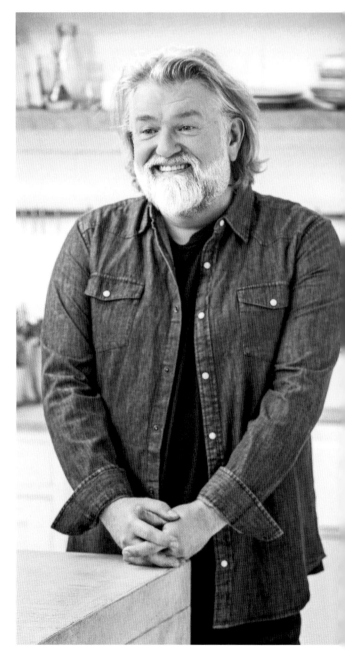

Dave

The hardest thing is when I'm working away from home and can't cook for myself. In these situations, I can end up grabbing something high-fat, quick and tasty. Then there's the doughnut in the car park syndrome – the snack we think doesn't count, but it does. For me, it's the scotch egg on the way out of the deli – something I scoff on the way home without really thinking about it. Fatal. I guess those sorts of snacks and takeaways can be the downfall for many of us, as you consume loads of calories without realising it. I have to make sure I have some healthy, low-calorie snacks available and also to not let myself get too hungry – then I'm far too easily tempted! Until I was about 50, I avoided getting on the scales – what the eye didn't see and all that. Now I weigh myself regularly because I know it's a whole lot easier to lose a few pounds than a few stone.

Si.

I struggle to get a proper structure to my food intake. I start off with the best intentions and then life – and me – gets in the way. I'm sensible in that I cook everything from scratch and avoid processed foods, but then I know I'm over-generous with the olive oil because I love it, and I can't resist bread and butter. I try not to have butter in the house because if it's there I'll slather it on everything. Then there's alcohol. I don't drink to get drunk. I drink for the taste – particularly since the availability of great craft beers and natural wines. And, of course, after a couple of glasses my resolve tends to go out of the window and I want to go in the kitchen and stuff myself with carbs. It's all the harder because I live by myself and there's no one to say, 'Hold on – what are you doing?' I've also had problems since having Covid. I didn't have it that badly, but ever since, I've struggled with lack of energy and motivation. I know what I need to do and want to do but it's hard sometimes, and when I'm stressed or feeling low, I take comfort in food. Then I put on weight and I don't like it. I don't like the way I look and feel. So, writing this book has helped me start getting back into good habits and I know I'll be all the better for it.

A QUICK ROUND UP

Professor Roy Taylor is a leading expert on type 2 diabetes. In his work at Newcastle University, he has shown exactly how type 2 diabetes develops, and in the process discovered how it could be reversed. He showed how the old idea that type 2 diabetes was inevitably lifelong was completely wrong. This has revolutionised treatments, with his dietary advice leading to proper weight loss. Here are his key points on healthy eating and weight control.

- Strict dieting should be an episode, not a life sentence.

- Rapid weight loss over a two- or three-month spell is more successful than slow weight loss.

- It's fine to count calories if that works for you but there's no need to obsess over them.

- It's more important to watch your portions and keep moving.

- Avoid highly processed foods and ready meals and eat a good range of fresh foods.

- It's OK to eat full-fat yoghurt, cheese, butter and so on, but remember that fat is high in calories so don't overdo it.

- Don't worry if you don't want to eat breakfast – but if you do, avoid carb-heavy meals, like cereal.

- Avoid fruit juice and smoothies. Stick to whole fruit.

- Think of 'five insteads a day' rather than five a day.

- Reduce serving sizes of rice, pasta, etc. That's more important than going for brown/wholemeal.

A personal message from Prof Roy

You eat food, not diets. But the huge problem in our society today is the flood of relatively inexpensive processed foods that pack in the calories but do not satisfy hunger for long. The type of food determines how many calories slip in each day. Many folk suffer the effects of being heavier than their own body wants them to be. But health issues can be dramatically affected by weight loss – from back pain, arthritis and heartburn, to the risk of weight-related cancers, premature heart trouble, blood pressure and diabetes. And that means finding a way that suits you of taking in fewer food calories.

Let's not beat around the bush: health is the number one component of happiness.

OUR NEW BOOK

Using Roy's advice, we've come up with more than 80 tasty new recipes for this book which is about eating for good health as well as losing weight. If you're in a weight-loss phase, take a look at the dishes in our 'Light low-cal' section. If you're looking to maintain a healthy weight, you can add some healthy sides to these or look at dishes in our 'Hearty but healthy' chapter.

START THE DAY RIGHT

Prof Roy says that a big carb load is the worst way to start the day. If you are a breakfast or brunch fan, these recipes will get you off to a good start with some dishes that are packed with flavour and protein but not too carb heavy, plus some healthy bread. Who can resist the thought of Turkish eggs or crumpets topped with smashed avocado?

LIGHT LOW-CAL MEALS

These low-calorie dishes are ideal when you are in a weight-loss phase, or you want a light meal to balance out your intake for the day. Recipes like our chicken and sweetcorn soup or cod and ham croquettes might be low in calories, but they are still spot on in terms of taste and interest.

SOMETHING TO SNACK ON

We all want a snack sometimes and this chapter is full of ideas for little treats to have on hand when the munchy moments strike – Marmite breadsticks anyone? We've come up with recipes for delicious dips to have on standby in the fridge and ideas for sandwich fillings to cheer up your lunch box.

HEARTY BUT HEALTHY

These recipes are higher in calories but still have a reasonably low fat and carb count, so are just the job for maintaining a good weight. As always, we've made sure that as well as being healthy they are tasty, tempting and lots of fun. Try our chicken and white bean chilli or settle down to a fab bowl of meatballs with curry sauce and know that your creation is doing you good, as well as giving your taste buds a treat.

A TOUCH OF SWEETNESS

OK, life without any cake or the occasional pudding is hard, but we've found ways to make some of our favourites less calorific and lower in fat and sugar, while still tasting the business. Try our apple crumble with a deliciously light and crisp topping or our Mojito fruit salad, or whip up some mini malt loaves that contain no refined sugar but still satisfy a sweet tooth.

SIDES & BASICS

Finally, we've provided some ideas for healthy side dishes that you'll find useful to add to your meals, particularly when you're in a weight-maintenance phase. Try our celeriac or white bean mash recipes and experiment with gut-friendly basics like kimchi and kefir.

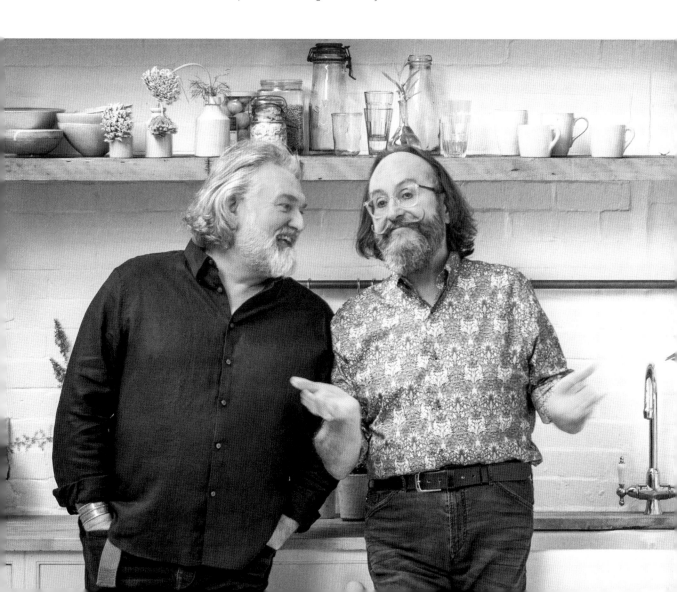

TOP TIPS FROM THE SUPER FIT!

When we were doing our research for this book, we also met up with an old friend who is one of the fittest people we know – said to have the best 'engine' in Britain – to get his take on healthy eating! Chris Thompson is an amazing Olympic marathon champion and he and his wife Jemma (who is also an Olympian) shared their health and dietary advice with us. They explained how athletes must learn to really listen to their body to achieve maximum fitness and health, and eating the right stuff is a crucial part of that. Chris admits that for a while when he was younger, he relied on his natural abilities and didn't think so much about what he put into his body. Jemma has been a great influence on his diet, helping him make sure that meals are enjoyable as well as a valuable part of their fitness regime.

While the rest of us might not have their superpowers, listening to your body and recognising the effects of different foods is helpful for us all. For Chris and Jemma, it is all about training, recovery and staying free of illness and injury, but their advice and experience also applies to anyone who wants to live a healthy and active lifestyle. This is what Chris told us about his and Jemma's regime.

- Start the day with some water – after all, the body has gone without all night. We both have a glass of water with a dash of lemon and a tiny pinch of salt first thing and always reach for a drink of water before opting for a snack. Often when you think you are hungry, you're actually just thirsty. Have a drink of water first and if that satisfies you, you know you were dehydrated. If not, you know you need to eat. Little things like that are important.

- Hydration is super-important for a healthy body – you die of thirst before you die of hunger! You need water in order to store the energy from the food you eat – otherwise it gets stored as fat. Water keeps everything in the body functioning more efficiently, including your digestion and bowels.

- Breakfast – everyone has different needs. If you're sitting most of the day, some protein and not too much in the way of carbs should suit you. If you're going to be more active, scale up your breakfast accordingly. We're both big fans of kefir, which is a fermented milk drink, a bit like thin yoghurt. It's believed to support the immune system and boost gut health as well as many other benefits. We have some every morning and we find it hugely beneficial to our general health. We prefer to make our own kefir rather than buy it – it's easy - and there's a recipe on page 177 of this book.

- Try to plan your food for the day or the week and you're more likely to make healthy choices. We have what we call our first-aid food kit in the freezer – healthy meals that we've batch-cooked and stashed away for the times when we get home tired and hungry after a long day and the last thing we want to think about is what to cook. That way we're not tempted to call for a takeaway. Planning ahead stops us from comfort eating and helps us keep to a balanced diet through the week. We also cook extra sometimes, so there are leftovers and we don't have to cook every night.

- Good planning applies to snacks as well. When you're out and about it can be hard to find healthy options and you might grab the quickest thing you can find. We try to keep some nourishing snacks, such as nuts and fresh fruit, on hand and we avoid having unhealthy stuff in the house too often – if it's not there you can't eat it! We also avoid going food shopping when hungry, as we're more likely to make poor choices. Listen to your body and think about what it needs, rather than giving in to your mind which is where the cravings for the wrong stuff hide.

- Listening to your body is important for everyone – not just athletes. Once you start eating better and more healthily, you'll become aware of changes in your skin and hair as well as your energy levels. Notice how you feel if one day you drink too much alcohol or overdo the sweet stuff. Recognise when you feel full and stop yourself reaching for a second helping out of habit.

- Watch for the triggers that make you reach for the wrong foods. Athletes are constantly undergoing the stress of training, but everyone deals with stress on a daily basis – whether it's not sleeping well or having too much pressure at work. Stress on your body comes in all sorts of ways, including from what you consume, such as processed foods, excess salt, sugar and alcohol. Because as athletes we're very tuned in to how our bodies feel, we really notice when we consume alcohol that's full of sugar and we often find we sleep less well. Poor-quality sleep or lack of sleep can also be a cause of weight gain, so it's important to try to create good sleeping habits.

- A nourishing dinner sets you up for the next day. We try to eat at least two or three hours before going to bed so the body has time to digest the food properly. And we know that if we eat late or have too much sugar or alcohol it affects not only our sleep but also how we feel the next day. Eating a good meal can act like a good training session – eat a meal with plenty of veg, some protein and high-fibre carbs and you'll feel better for it the next day and have more energy. What's more, it's easier to make good decisions when rested and healthy. When you're stressed and tired, you're more likely to make bad food choices.

- Keep a check on yourself and try not to just reach for treats like a chocolate bar or a glass of wine without thinking. It might de-stress your mind in the moment but not your body. If you look to healthier options, this will very quickly reward your body and will positively affect your mindset too – good habits breed good habits.

- Pick smart moments to have treats like wine or favourite foods, so that the knock-on effect doesn't bring about more stress and the desire for more 'treats'. For instance, too many midweek treats can have an impact on the next working day. Eat to perform well at work and find time to treat yourself when you can rest.

- Finally, none of us are perfect. Even Olympic athletes. If we manage to make the right choices 70 or 80 per cent of the time, we reckon we're doing well. Just try to do your best and forgive yourself for the lapses. If you have a bad day's eating, make up for it the next day by having healthy meals that are delicious and good for you. Keep that health scale tipped in your favour.

NUTRITIONAL INFO

Full nutritional info is given for each recipe. Unless otherwise noted, the figures are per serving, without any extras. Quantities are in grams. Anything less than 0.5 grams of salt is listed as a trace.

Calories measure the amount of energy in the food. It can be tedious and not necessary to count calories every day, but it's useful to know the dangerous calorie-bomb foods. Everyone should know the approximate number of calories in the food they eat.

Protein helps you feel satisfied, and we need protein to maintain our body's processes. Nuts and pulses, as well as meat, fish, eggs and dairy, are all good sources.

Carbohydrates are made up of lots of sugar molecules bound together. Your digestion will turn them into sugar. But some are digested faster than others – and slowly digested carbs, like wholegrain foods, are easier for your body to handle. The huge problem is added sugar in highly processed foods, such as ready meals and takeaways. By avoiding processed foods, you'll benefit more than by worrying about different types of carbs.

Sugar – figures listed are for the total sugar in a dish, which includes the natural sugars in fruit, vegetables and dairy. It is the added sugar or free sugar, like the sugar added to tea or used in puddings, that we need to limit and keep as low as possible for weight loss and good health.

Fat – this figure is the total fat contained in a serving (monounsaturated, polyunsaturated and saturated). Monounsaturated fat – in foods such as nuts, seeds and olive oil – and polyunsaturated fats in oily fish are better for you than saturated fat but still high in calories. Fats are made up of strings of carbon atoms with lots of energy stored in the links between them. Gram for gram they are the most calorie-dense food.

Saturated fats have different links between the carbon atoms (they are 'saturated' with hydrogen atoms). They are less healthy inside the body, but most people – even experts – don't realise that any excess carbohydrate is turned into 100 per cent saturated fat in the body, whereas butter is only around 50 per cent saturated fat. The total amount of food eaten matters more than the type of fat in food.

Fibre is not digested and so does not add calories. It is contained in plant foods, such as fruit, vegetables, nuts and seeds, as well as in grains and we need a good amount of fibre in the diet to help digestion. Wholegrain bread, brown rice and brown pasta contain more fibre than refined varieties.

Salt – The figures given are for the salt content in the ingredients, not any extra added to taste.

A few notes from us

- Follow the recipes carefully so you don't change the calorie count or nutritional details. Weigh your ingredients and use proper measuring spoons and a measuring jug.

- We've made oven temperatures as accurate as possible, but all ovens are different, so keep an eye on your dish and be prepared to cook it for a longer or shorter time if necessary.

- Use free-range eggs whenever possible. We generally use large eggs unless otherwise specified.

- Peel vegetables, onions and garlic unless otherwise specified.

- Home-made stock is great to have in the freezer, so we've included a few recipes. But if you don't have time, you'll find good fresh stocks in the supermarket or use cubes or those little stock pots.

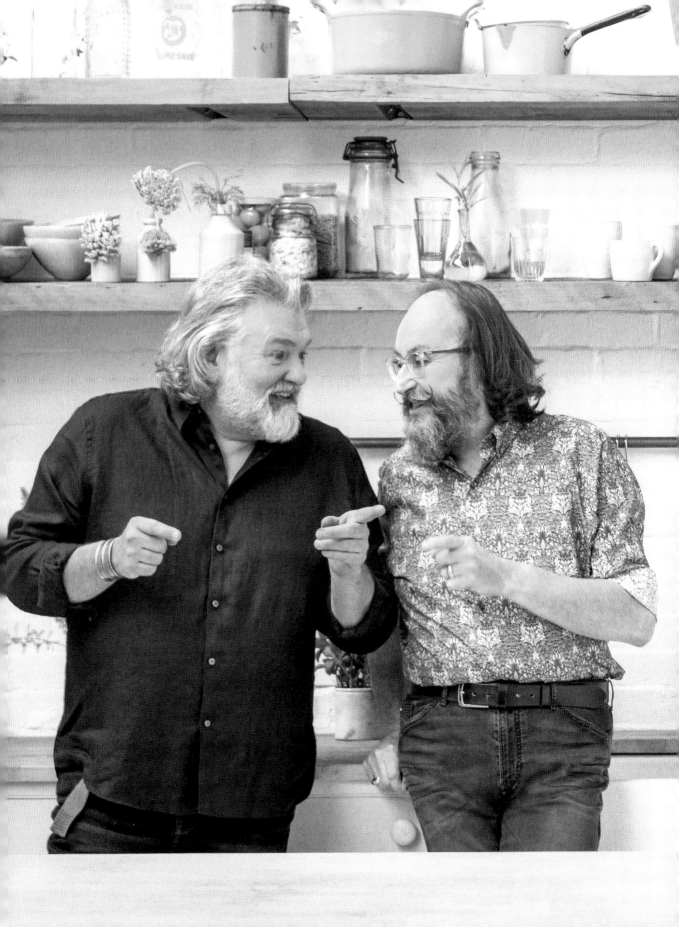

START
DAY

THE RIGHT

SMASHED AVOCADO ON CRUMPETS

zest and juice of ½ lemon
1 small red onion, very finely
    chopped
2 large or 3 small avocados,
    peeled and stoned
leaves from 2 mint sprigs,
    finely chopped
generous pinch of chilli powder
8 crumpets
½ tsp smoked chilli flakes
black sesame seeds
4 tsp pomegranate molasses
sea salt

We're both big fans of crumpets and they're not too high in calories if you don't slather them in loads of butter. We've giving them a bit of an update with this recipe which really packs a punch. A hit of chilli helps to wake you up in the morning and this breakfast treat takes very little effort to put together.

Put the lemon zest and juice into a bowl and add the red onion and some salt. Leave to marinate for up to half an hour – this will take some of the bitterness out of the onion.

Add the avocados and mash them roughly, then stir in the mint and chill powder.

Toast the crumpets and top each one with a generous amount of the avocado mixture. Sprinkle with chilli flakes and sesame seeds, then drizzle with pomegranate molasses – a scant half teaspoon per crumpet. Serve immediately while the crumpets are still hot.

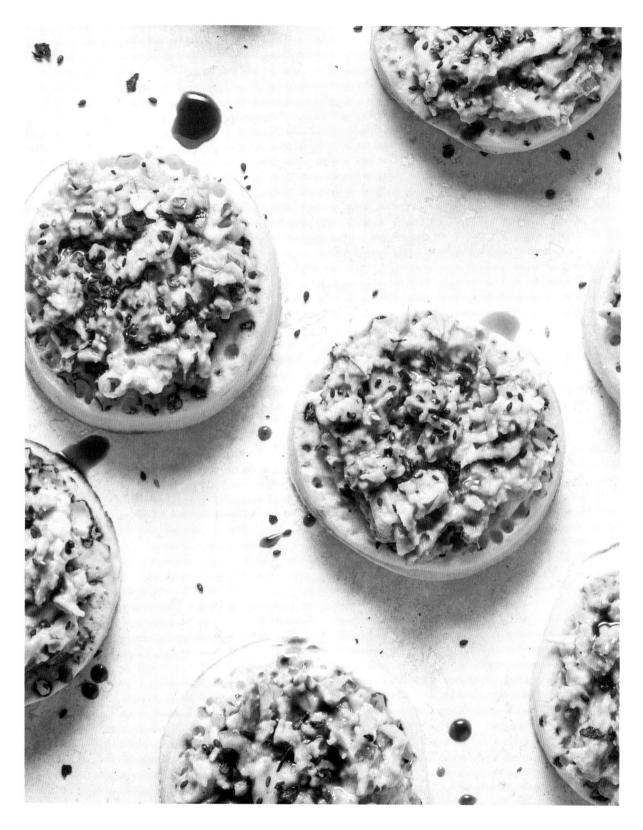

INFO PER SERVING (2 CRUMPETS):   CALORIES 454   PROTEIN (G) 9.5   CARBS (G) 50   SUGAR (G) 9
FAT (G) 22.5   SATURATED FAT (G) 4.5   FIBRE (G) 8.5   SALT (G) 1.2

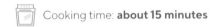
EGGS FLORENTINE

450g spinach
squeeze of lemon juice
1 tsp white wine vinegar
4 eggs
2 muffins, split (optional)

Béarnaise sauce
2 large tarragon sprigs
1 shallot, finely chopped
50ml white wine or vermouth
1 tbsp white wine vinegar
100ml crème fraiche
2 egg yolks
½ tsp Dijon mustard
a few chives, finely chopped
squeeze of lemon juice (optional)
sea salt and black pepper

Eggs are a great breakfast choice as they are high in protein and really keep you satisfied. Up to you whether you opt for the muffins – they up your carb count but do provide some fibre and bulk. The sauce is totally delicious and there's no need for cornflour or any other thickener, as the mustard and egg yolks do the job.

First make the sauce. Strip the leaves from the tarragon sprigs and chop them finely, then set aside. Roughly chop the stems and add them to a small saucepan with the shallot, white wine or vermouth and the vinegar. Bring to the boil, boil for 1 minute, then remove the pan from the heat. Leave to infuse until cool.

Strain the liquid through a sieve, then tip it back into the pan and add the crème fraiche. Heat it through, then season with salt and pepper and beat in the egg yolks and mustard. Add the tarragon leaves and the chives. Taste for seasoning and acidity and add a squeeze of lemon juice if you like, then whisk briskly until the sauce is aerated. Keep warm and whisk again before serving.

Wash the spinach thoroughly and shake off any excess water. Put it in a saucepan and season with salt and pepper. Set the pan over a high heat and keep pressing the spinach with a spoon until it has wilted completely. Season with a squeeze of lemon juice, then drain in a colander, gently squeezing to remove excess water.

To poach the eggs, bring a saucepan of water to the boil and add the vinegar. Lower the eggs, still in their shells, into the water and leave foR 20 seconds exactly, then remove.

Turn the heat down to a simmer. Swirl the water to create a whirlpool effect and carefully crack the eggs into the water, one at a time. Cook for 3 minutes, then remove with a slotted spoon and place on some kitchen towel to drain.

Serve the eggs on the spinach, drizzle over the sauce and season with black pepper. If using muffins, toast them lightly , top with spinach and add the eggs and sauce.

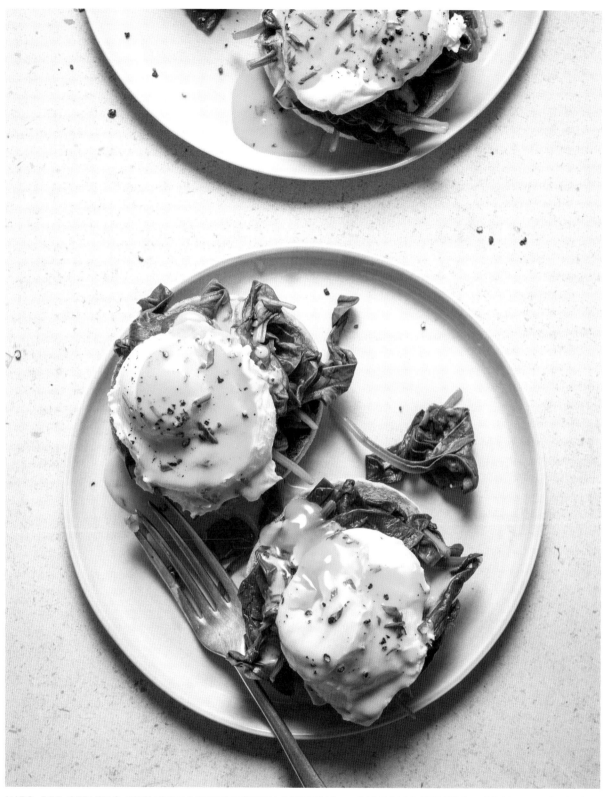

INFO PER SERVING WITHOUT MUFFINS/WITH MUFFINS: CALORIES 365/530   PROTEIN (G) 23/30
CARBS (G) 2/32   SUGAR (G) 1.5/4   FAT (G) 27/28   SATURATED FAT (G) 15/28   FIBRE (G) 2.5/17
SALT (G) 0.8/1.5

BREAKFAST TRAY BAKE

1 onion, cut into wedges

1 large red pepper, cut into strips

1 sweet potato, peeled and cut into cubes

2 tsp olive oil

4 sausages, skinned, halved and rolled into balls

12 chestnut mushrooms, left whole

4 medium tomatoes, halved

4 eggs

1 tsp dried sage

sea salt and black pepper

A great guilt-free way of enjoying a full English, this is a brilliant dish for a family breakfast. It's easy to prepare and contains a good amount of protein. If you like, you can also add little nests of spinach. Cubes of frozen spinach work well – just defrost them and shape them into rings, then drop an egg into each one.

Preheat the oven to 200°C/Fan 180°C/Gas 6.

Put the onion, red pepper and sweet potato in a large roasting tin. Drizzle over a teaspoon of the olive oil and mix thoroughly, then season with salt and pepper. Add the sausage balls and roast in the oven for 25 minutes.

Toss the mushrooms in the remaining oil and add them to the tin with the tomatoes. Roast for a further 5 minutes.

Make 4 dips in the veg and add the eggs. Sprinkle over the sage, season the eggs with a little salt and roast for a further 5 minutes. The egg whites should be just set and the yolks will be a mixture of runny and slightly fudgy. Serve at once.

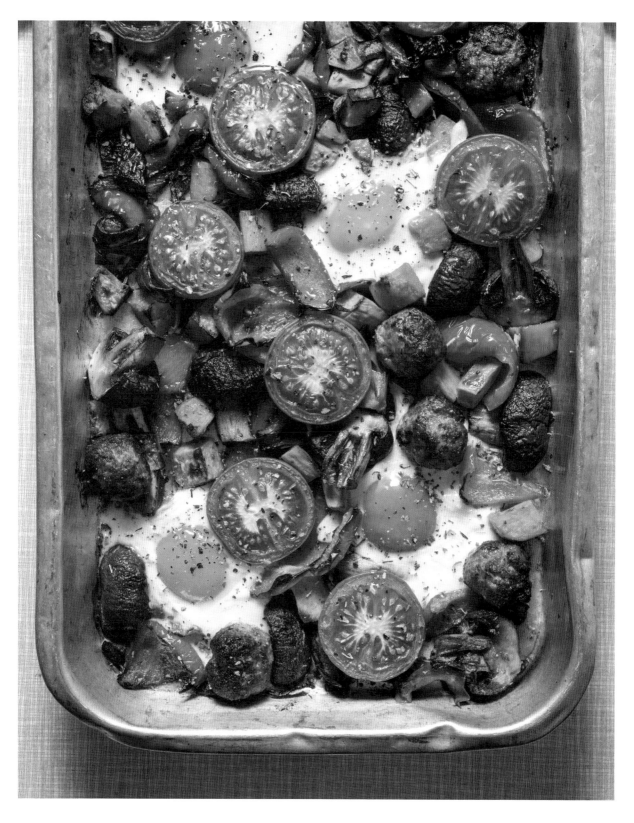

INFO PER SERVING: CALORIES 341   PROTEIN (G) 18   CARBS (G) 19   SUGAR (G) 10.5   FAT (G) 20
SATURATED FAT (G) 7   FIBRE (G) 5   SALT (G) 1.1

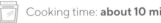
TURKISH EGGS

Yoghurt
150g yoghurt or thick kefir
1 small garlic clove, crushed
    (optional)
zest of ½ lemon
sea salt

Chilli oil
1 tbsp olive oil
1 tsp butter
½ tsp paprika
½ tsp chilli flakes

To serve
1 tsp white wine vinegar
2–4 fresh eggs
juice of ½ lemon
leaves from a few parsley sprigs,
    finely chopped

Here's our Turkish de-light! This popular Turkish breakfast dish makes a nice change from regular poached eggs and we've reduced the calories in our new version. You don't have to heat the yoghurt like we suggest, but it is a good way of bringing the temperature up, making the dish even nicer to eat. It helps to mellow the garlic, too. Up to you whether you serve this with one or two eggs per person – we like two.

First prepare the yoghurt or kefir. Put it in a heatproof bowl with the garlic, if using, the lemon zest and a pinch of salt. Set the bowl over a saucepan of simmering water and whisk the yoghurt or kefir as it heats. The aim is to get it to blood temperature. Remove the bowl from the heat, cover and set aside while you prepare the eggs and oil.

To prepare the oil, heat the olive oil and butter in a small saucepan until the butter has melted. Add the paprika and chilli flakes and swirl around to combine. Season with salt.

To poach the eggs, bring a saucepan of water to the boil and add the vinegar. Lower the eggs, still in their shells, into the water and leave for 20 seconds exactly, then remove.

Turn the heat down to a simmer. Swirl the water to create a whirlpool effect and carefully crack the eggs into the water, one at a time. Cook for 3 minutes, then remove with a slotted spoon and place on some kitchen paper to drain.

To assemble, divide the yoghurt or kefir between 2 shallow bowls and top with the eggs. Drizzle over the chilli oil, then squeeze over the lemon juice and garnish with the parsley.

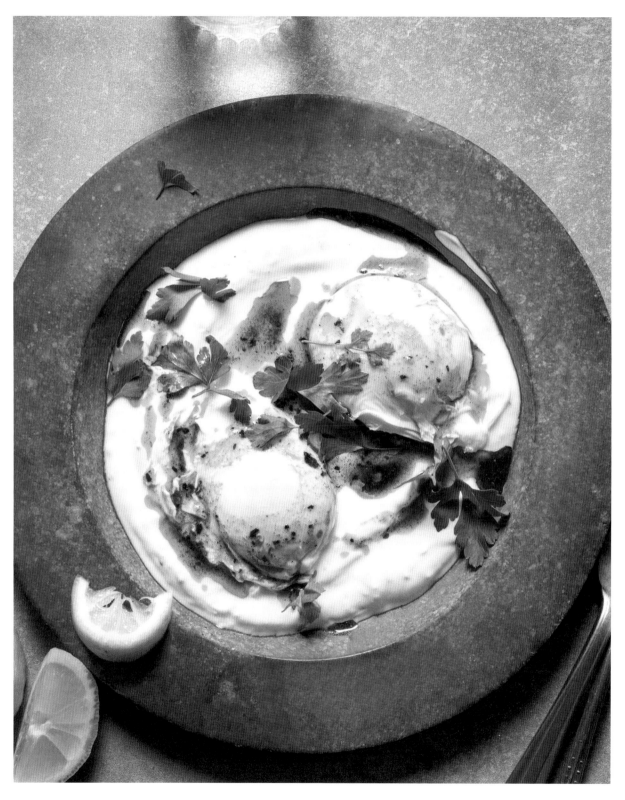

INFO PER SERVING WITH 1 EGG/WITH 2 EGGS: CALORIES 208/288   PROTEIN (G) 12/20   CARBS (G) 5.5/5.5   SUGAR (G) 5.5/5.5   FAT (G) 15/20   SATURATED FAT (G) 5/6.5   FIBRE (G) O/O SALT (G) TRACE/O.7

SYRNIKI PANCAKES

50g raisins
juice and zest of ½ large orange
300g quark
200g full-fat cottage cheese,
    drained
35g caster sugar
2 eggs
50g plain flour
pinch of salt
oil or butter, for frying
plain yoghurt, for serving
    (optional)

Blueberry compote
250g blueberries
1 tsp honey
zest and juice of ½ orange

We first discovered these tasty little treats when we were filming a television series in the Baltic a few years ago. They're a traditional dish and can be quite rich, but we've lightened up our recipe by reducing the sugar and flour and using more quark than cottage cheese. The pancakes are soft, tasty and comforting and good just as they are or served with blueberry compote. If you like, you can make the pancakes ahead of time and wrap them in foil, ready to pop in a warm oven to reheat when you're ready to eat.

First put the raisins and orange juice in a small saucepan and bring to the boil. Remove from the heat and leave until the raisins have absorbed all the liquid.

Put the quark and cottage cheese in a large bowl and beat to remove the lumps from the cottage cheese. Add the orange zest, sugar, eggs and flour with a pinch of salt and mix thoroughly. You could also do this in a food processor. Stir in the soaked raisins and leave the batter to rest for at least half an hour. If you want to get ahead, it's fine to make the batter in advance and chill it for several hours or overnight.

When you are ready to make the pancakes, heat a large frying pan. Add a few drops of oil or a tiny knob of butter, then rub over the pan with kitchen paper. Dot dessertspoons of the batter over the frying pan – you should manage to make about 5 at a time.

Cook the pancakes until bubbles appear on the surface and they are starting to look set around the edges. They should come away cleanly and be a dappled golden brown. Flip over and cook until they are golden brown on the other side. Repeat until you have cooked all the pancakes.

To make the compote, put the blueberries in a small pan with the honey, orange zest and juice. Heat gently until most of the blueberries have burst and the liquid looks syrupy. Serve with the pancakes.

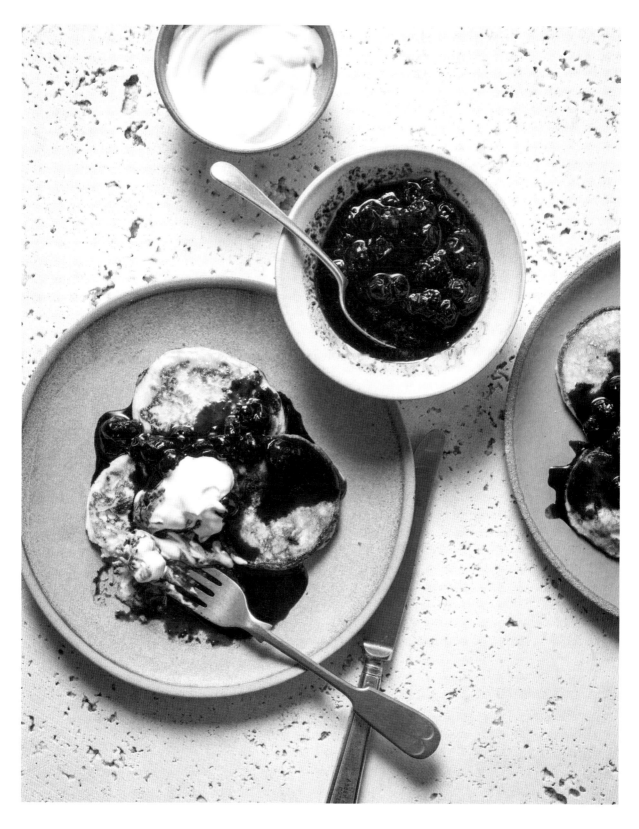

INFO PER SERVING OF 6 PANCAKES AND COMPOTE: CALORIES 325   PROTEIN (G) 22   CARBS (G) 39
SUGAR (G) 29   FAT (G) 9   SATURATED FAT (G) 3   FIBRE (G) 1.5   SALT (G) 0.8

SAUSAGE & BACON ROOT VEG HASH

75g smoked bacon, finely diced

2 sausages (about 150g in weight), skinned

1 large onion, finely chopped

800g root vegetables – any combination of potato (unpeeled), carrot, celeriac, swede, parsnip, turnip or Jerusalem artichoke, all diced into 1cm cubes

1 tbsp Worcestershire sauce

1 tbsp brown sauce

1 tbsp tomato ketchup

1 tsp dried sage

sea salt and black pepper

To serve (optional)

steamed greens

fried or poached eggs

Nothing like a good hash to start the day and this one is easy, as once you've done the initial browning you just pop it all in the oven to cook. No need to stand there stirring. We've used a little bit of meat to add flavour and give enough fat for cooking the veg. Choose whatever root vegetables you like, but we suggest keeping the amount of potato to 200g or less.

Preheat the oven to 200°C/Fan 180°C/Gas 6. Put the bacon, sausages and onion into a hot frying pan and cook until well browned, stirring regularly to break up the sausage meat. The bacon and sausage will provide enough fat, so you don't need to add more.

Put all the vegetables in a saucepan and cover them with water. Bring to the boil and cook for 2 minutes, then drain.

Put the fried bacon, sausage and onion into a large roasting tin with the vegetables. Mix the Worcestershire sauce, brown sauce and ketchup together with a tablespoon of water and the dried sage. Pour this mixture over the contents of the roasting tin and season with salt and pepper. Mix thoroughly.

Roast in the oven for about 30 minutes, stirring once or twice until the vegetables are knife tender and crisp around the edges. Serve with plenty of steamed greens and an egg on top, if you like.

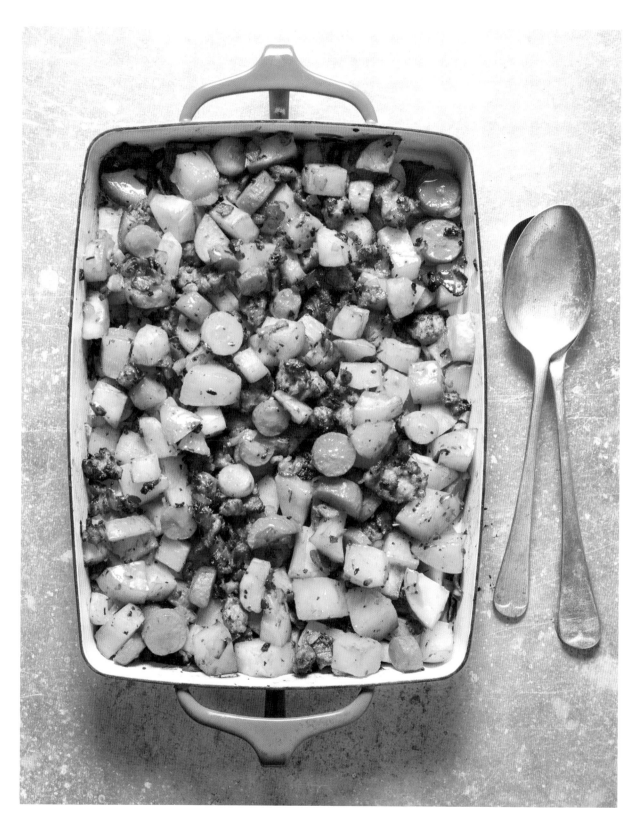

INFO PER SERVING/WITH FRIED EGG: CALORIES 283/403   PROTEIN (G) 12/20.5   CARBS (G) 27/27
SUGAR (G) 13/13   FAT (G) 12/21.5   SATURATED FAT (G) 4.5/6.5   FIBRE (G) 9/9   SALT (G) 1.6/1.85

CLOUD BREAD

3 eggs, separated
¼ tsp cream of tartar (optional)
50g quark or cream cheese
1 tsp apple cider vinegar
sea salt and black pepper

Optional extras
½ tsp garlic powder
¼ tsp ground turmeric
¼ tsp cayenne or other chilli
   powder
½ tsp dried herbs (oregano,
   mixed, thyme)
2 tsp poppy seeds
1 tbsp milled flax seeds
1 tsp finely chopped fresh herbs
   (coriander, parsley)

To garnish
2 tbsp finely grated Parmesan
   cheese
sesame, nigella, cumin or
   caraway seeds

This grain-free bread was a new one on us – it sounds kind of bonkers but it works. And if you're watching the carbs or avoiding gluten you'll love it. The recipe is amazingly versatile – you can make any size breads you like and add any flavours you fancy. We've suggested a good size to get you started, but you can pile the mixture up higher to make thicker pieces and cook them for a bit longer, or make them thinner to use as pizza bases or tortilla substitutes. Also, you can reheat the breads in a dry frying pan or in the oven.

Preheat the oven to 150°C/Fan 130°C/Gas 2. Line a couple of baking trays with baking parchment.

Put the egg whites in a bowl with the cream of tartar, if using, and whisk until they are very firm and dry. You should be able to turn the bowl upside down without the mixture dropping out.

Put the egg yolks and the quark or cream cheese in a separate bowl with salt and pepper, the vinegar and any of the optional extras you like. Beat until the mixture is smooth and no flecks of quark or cream cheese remain. Then carefully add a spoonful of the egg whites and fold it in until completely combined. Add the rest of the egg whites and fold them – try to avoid knocking out too much air.

Spoon rounds of the mixture on to the lined baking trays, spacing them out well. You can vary the sizes but dividing the mixture by 8 will give you rounds with a diameter of about 12cm with a depth of about 1cm. Sprinkle with cheese and/or seeds.

Bake in the preheated oven for about 20 minutes until golden brown with a cracked top. Remove the breads from the oven and carefully peel them away from the baking parchment. Leave to cool, then eat or store in the fridge.

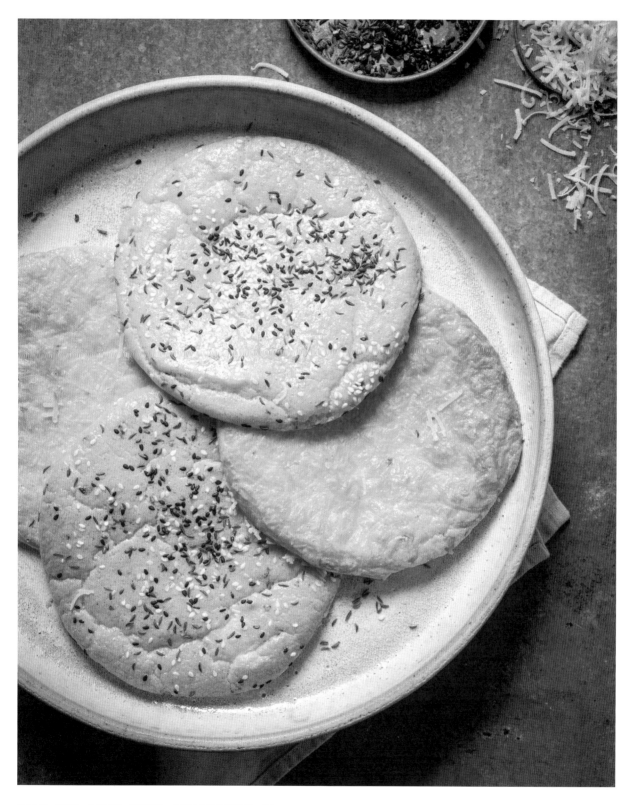

INFO PER PIECE WITH QUARK/WITH CREAM CHEESE: CALORIES 50/60 PROTEIN (G) 5/4.5 CARBS (G) 0.5/0.3 SUGAR (G) 0.5/0.3 FAT (G) 3/4.5 SATURATED FAT (G) 1.5/2.5 FIBRE (G) 0/0 SALT (G) TRACE/TRACE

SAVOURY APPLE MUFFINS

300g wholemeal flour

2 tsp baking powder

½ tsp bicarbonate of soda

1 tsp dried sage

30g pumpkin seeds

pinch of salt

300ml buttermilk

60ml olive oil

2 eggs

2 large eating apples, peeled
and finely chopped or grated

75g hard cheese such as Cheddar,
grated

A muffin makes a good option for a breakfast snack on the go. These are satisfyingly savoury but with a touch of sweetness from the apple – just what you need. You could also make smaller ones in fairy cake tins if you like. A clever little number, we reckon.

Preheat the oven to 200°C/Fan 180°C/Gas 6. Line a 12-hole muffin tin with cases or lightly oil the holes.

Mix the flour, baking powder, bicarb, sage and pumpkin seeds together with a good pinch of salt. Then whisk the buttermilk, oil and eggs together in a large bowl and stir in the apples and cheese. Add the flour mixture and stir, keeping the mixing to a minimum.

Spoon the mixture into the muffin tin – you should have enough for about 2 tablespoons per hole.

Bake in the oven for 15–20 minutes until the muffins are well risen and golden brown. Leave them to cool and store in an airtight tin.

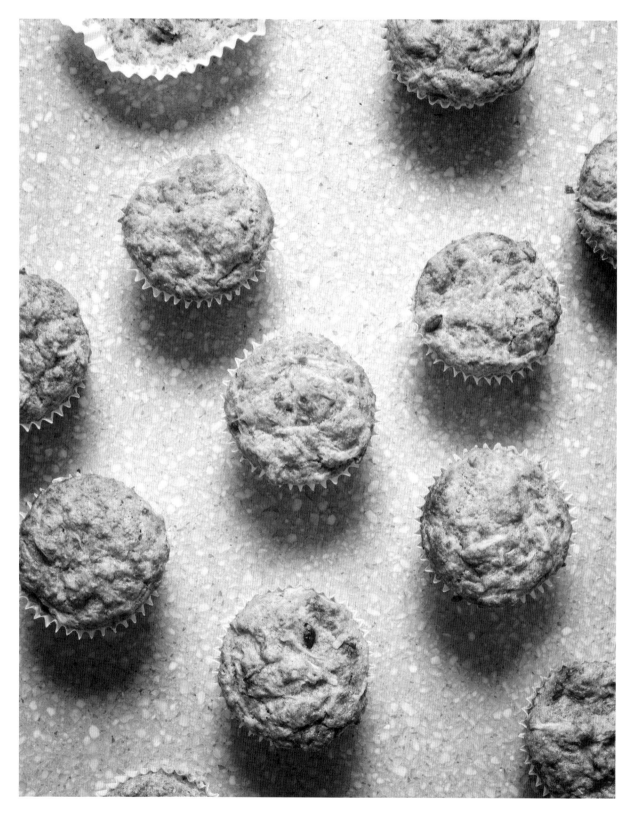

INFO PER MUFFIN: CALORIES 200   PROTEIN (G) 7   CARBS (G) 21   SUGAR (G) 4.5   FAT (G) 8.5
SATURATED FAT (G) 2.5   FIBRE (G) 3   SALT (G) 0.6

FOUR-SEED BREAD

500g malted grain flour, plus
   extra for dusting

7g fast-action dried yeast

8g salt

25g pumpkin seeds

25g sunflower seeded

25g milled flax seeds

15g sesame seeds

25ml olive or rapeseed oil

1 tsp honey

300ml warm water

There's something so nice about home-made bread – starting with the smell of it baking! And the great thing is you know exactly what's in it and you know it's healthy. Packed with highly nutritious seeds, this recipe offers you a bit extra – so use your loaf and have a go. You can buy multi-seed flour, available in supermarkets, if you like, instead of using individual types of seeds.

Put the flour in a large bowl and mix in the yeast. Add the salt and seeds, then drizzle in the oil and honey. Slowly work in the warm water until you have a fairly sticky dough. Cover and leave to stand for half an hour.

Dust a work surface with flour and turn out the dough. Knead until it is soft and very elastic, then try the windowpane test. To do this, break off a small piece of dough and stretch it out until it is so thin you can almost see through it. If you can do this, the gluten has developed enough and the dough is ready, but if the dough breaks, knead it for longer. If you prefer, you can knead the dough in a stand mixer.

Put the dough back in the bowl and cover with a damp cloth. Leave to stand for a couple of hours until doubled in size.

Knock back the dough until it deflates, then give it another quick knead and shape it into an oblong to fit into a large (900g) loaf tin. Cover with a damp cloth and leave to rise again. Preheat the oven to its highest setting.

When the dough has risen and has a well-rounded, springy dome, put it in the oven. Bake for about 25 minutes, then take it out and check it has a crisp, well-browned exterior and a hollow-sounding bottom. If you feel the base needs crisping up, pop the loaf back in the oven without the tin for a further 5 minutes. Leave to cool covered with a tea towel to maintain a perfect crisp, but not too hard, crust.

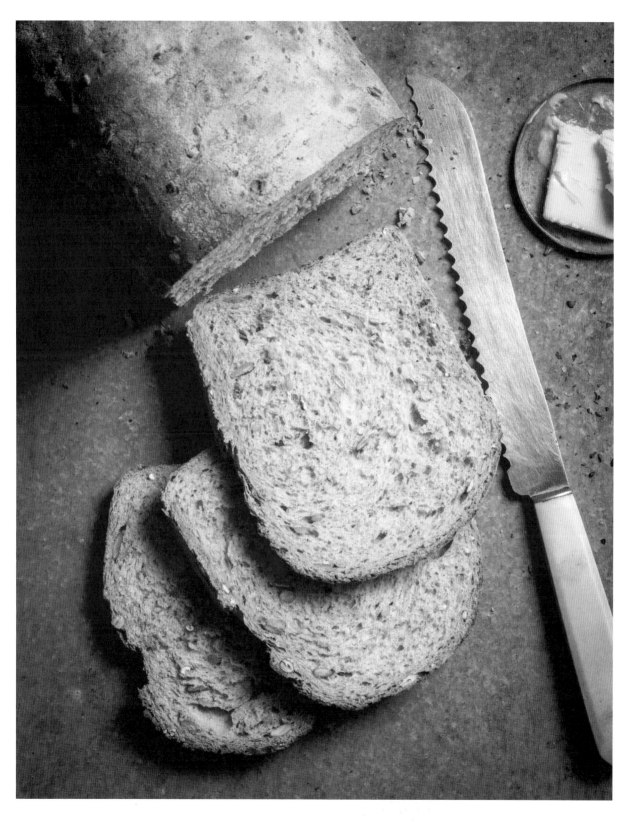

INFO PER SLICE (12 SLICES):   CALORIES 202   PROTEIN (G) 8   CARBS (G) 27   SUGAR (G) 1.2   FAT (G) 5.5
SATURATED FAT (G) 0.8   FIBRE (G) 4   SALT (G) 0.6

LIGHT
CALM

LOW-

EALS

THREE-LENTIL SOUP

50g yellow split peas, soaked
    overnight
50g brown or green lentils,
    well rinsed
50g split red lentils, well rinsed
1.2 litres ham, chicken or
    vegetable stock
1 tbsp tomato purée
1 onion, peeled and halved
1 bouquet garni made up of
    2 bay leaves, 1 thyme sprig,
    a few allspice berries and
    2 cloves
1 garlic bulb, left whole
sea salt and black pepper

Garnish
1 tsp olive oil
50g ham, shredded
1 tbsp maple syrup
pinch of chilli powder

Keep your finger on the pulse and try this! Using three different sorts of lentils gives the soup a nice range of textures and tastes and it's simple to prepare as there is no chopping or sautéing. For the garnish, use meat from a cooked ham rather than slices if possible, as it can be pulled into shreds more easily.

Drain the split peas and put them with the brown or green lentils and the red lentils in a large saucepan. Cover with the stock, bring to the boil and boil fiercely for 10 minutes.

Stir in the tomato purée until it has dissolved into the cooking liquid, then add the onion halves and the bouquet garni. Rub off the papery outer layers of the garlic bulb and add it to the pan too. Season with salt and pepper.

Bring back to the boil, then turn the heat down to a simmer and partially cover the pan. Simmer for up to an hour until the lentils are tender. The red lentils should have completely broken down and thickened the soup, while the split peas and the green or brown lentils should still be intact.

Fish out the bouquet garni, onion halves and the garlic. Squeeze out the flesh of the garlic and put it back in the pan. Roughly mash the onion and add this too. Check for seasoning and serve the soup piping hot.

For the garnish, heat the olive oil in a frying pan and add the ham. Drizzle over the maple syrup and season with salt, pepper and the chilli powder. Fry until the ham looks well caramelised, then sprinkle some over each serving of soup.

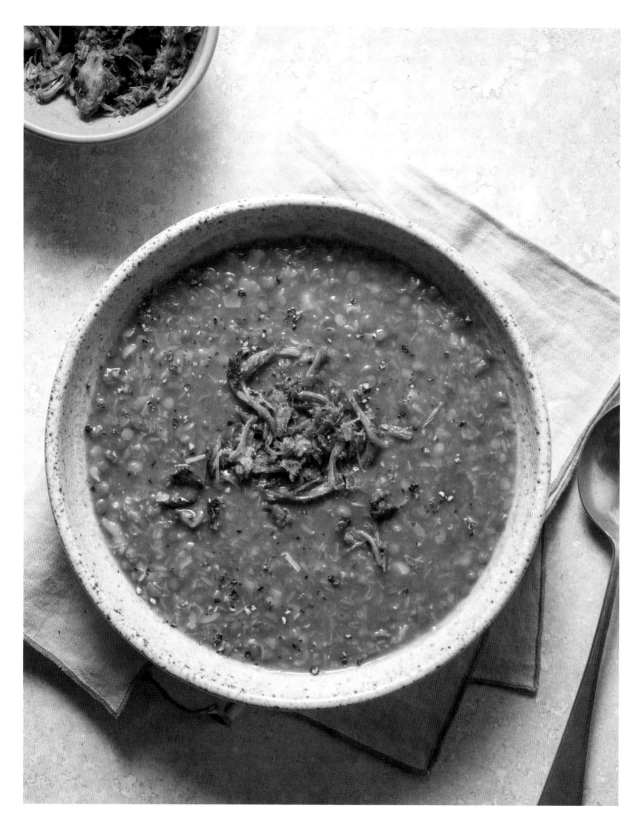

INFO PER SERVING: CALORIES 226   PROTEIN (G) 20   CARBS (G) 29   SUGAR (G) 7.5   FAT (G) 2.5
SATURATED FAT (G) 0.7   FIBRE (G) 5   SALT (G) 0.7

LEEK, CELERY & PARSLEY SOUP

15g olive oil or butter
1 large onion, finely chopped
2 leeks, finely sliced
2 celery sticks, finely chopped
150g floury potato, diced
small bunch of parsley, stems
   and leaves divided, chopped
1 litre chicken or vegetable stock
sea salt and black pepper

A good tasty soup is an ideal option when you're watching the calories, as it makes a warming, nourishing meal that feels satisfying but is low-cal. Adding a little potato means this is deliciously creamy, so you don't need to add any milk or cream. It's simple but full of flavour.

Heat the olive oil or butter in a large saucepan. Add all the vegetables and sauté for several minutes until the onion, leeks and celery start to look translucent and the pieces of potato are becoming rough around the edges.

Season well with salt and pepper and stir in the parsley stems. Pour in the stock and bring to the boil. Reduce the heat to a simmer and partially cover the pan. Leave to simmer for about 20 minutes until the vegetables are tender.

Blitz the soup until smooth, using a stick or jug blender. Add the chopped parsley leaves and blitz again until the soup is evenly flecked with green. Serve piping hot.

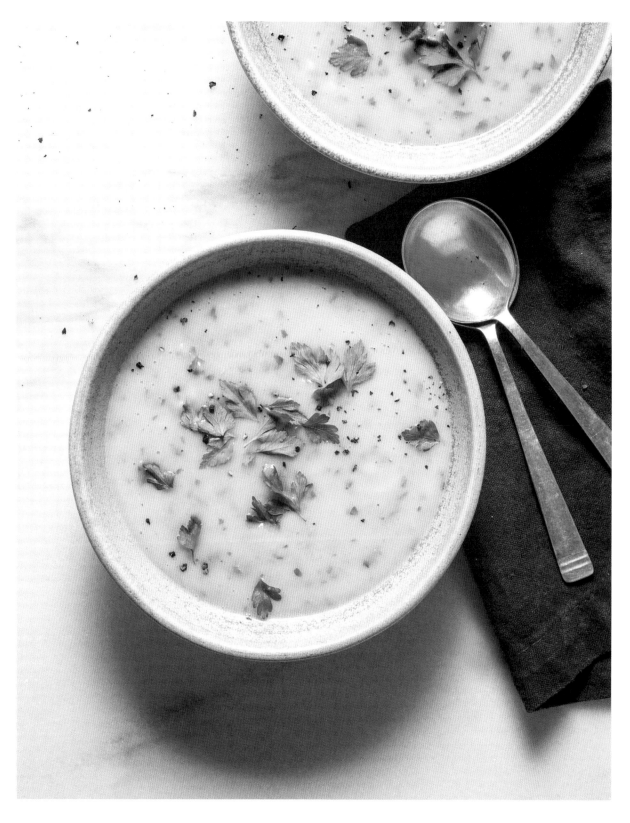

INFO PER SERVING: CALORIES 137   PROTEIN (G) 9   CARBS (G) 14.5   SUGAR (G) 6   FAT (G) 3.5
SATURATED FAT (G) 1   FIBRE (G) 5   SALT (G) 0.4

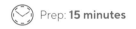
CHILLED WATERMELON SOUP

1 large cucumber
300g watermelon, peeled and
    roughly chopped (prepared
    weight)
300g tomatoes, roughly chopped
5g root ginger, finely chopped
1 small garlic clove, finely chopped
2 spring onions, cut into rounds
2 celery sticks, roughly chopped
juice of 1 orange
½ tsp hot paprika
sea salt and black pepper

To serve
juice of ½ lime
1–2 tsp sherry vinegar
ice cubes
100g feta cheese, crumbled
2 tbsp pumpkin seeds
drizzle of olive oil

Slightly sweet, slightly savoury, this is a very refreshing version of gazpacho, with a hint of heat from the ginger and paprika. It makes a perfect lunch on a hot day and the watermelon works really well with the feta cheese. Trust us on this – it's magnificent.

Top and tail the cucumber and peel it, then cut it in half lengthways and remove the seeds. Roughly chop the flesh. Put the cucumber, watermelon, tomatoes, ginger, garlic, spring onions, celery, orange juice and paprika into a blender with salt and black pepper. Blitz until smooth, then for extra smoothness, pass the mixture through a sieve. Chill until ready to serve.

Before serving, stir in the lime juice and add the sherry vinegar a few drops at a time. Keep tasting until you are satisfied you have got the balance right. If serving the soup at the table, add a few ice cubes to keep it chilled.

Top with some feta, a few pumpkin seeds and a drizzle of olive oil.

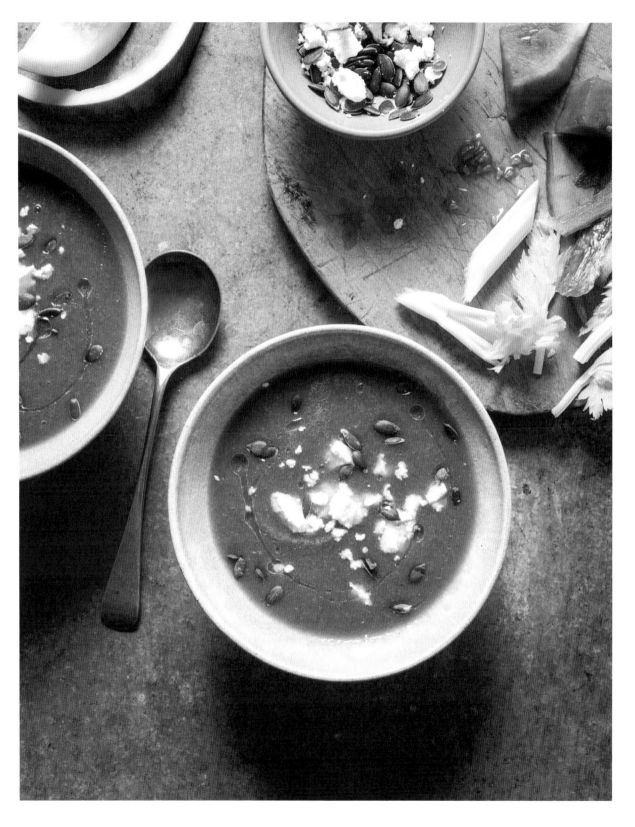

INFO PER SERVING: CALORIES 192   PROTEIN (G) 7.5   CARBS (G) 12   SUGAR (G) 11   FAT (G) 12
SATURATED FAT (G) 4.5   FIBRE (G) 2.5   SALT (G) 0.7

FISH BALL SOUP

Broth

1.5 litres chicken, fish or veg stock
15g root ginger, thinly sliced
4 garlic cloves, bruised
2 lemongrass stalks, bruised
2 bird's-eye chillies, pierced with
    the tip of a knife
4 fresh lime leaves, finely sliced
2 tsp light soft brown sugar
2 tbsp fish sauce
zest and juice of 1 lime

Fish balls

2 fresh lime leaves, shredded
2 garlic cloves, finely chopped
1 tbsp chopped coriander stems
1 tbsp fish sauce
400g white fish fillets, skinned
    and diced
1 egg white
1 tbsp rice flour or cornflour
sea salt and black or white pepper

To serve

200g sprouting broccoli
100g baby corn, halved
    lengthways
1 red pepper, sliced into strips
1 courgette, cut into rounds
100g bean sprouts
3 spring onions, cut into rounds
coriander sprigs
lime wedges

This makes a superb low-cal option if you're on a diet, but if you're not watching your weight and just want something healthy and delicious, you could add 150g of rice noodles. Try to get hold of some fresh lime leaves if you possibly can, as they do add to the flavour. Dried ones aren't as good. And we have to say – making your own fish balls really is worth the effort.

First make the broth. Put the stock and all the aromatics into a large saucepan and bring to the boil. Reduce to a simmer, cover and cook for 10 minutes. Leave to infuse until you are ready to use it.

Strain the broth through a sieve into a clean pan, reheat, then taste. Season and add more sugar, fish sauce or lime juice to taste.

To make the fish balls, put the lime leaves, garlic and coriander into a small food processor with the fish sauce. Process until broken down to a paste, then add the fish, egg white and rice flour or cornflour. Season with salt and plenty of black or white pepper. Blitz until the fish is well broken down and the mixture clumps together.

Divide the fish mixture into 12 balls and flatten them slightly. Put them in the fridge to chill until needed.

Add the sprouting broccoli, baby corn, red pepper and courgette to the reheated broth. Simmer for 3–4 minutes, then add the fish balls. Simmer for a further 5 minutes until the fish balls are just cooked through.

Divide the fish balls and vegetables between 4 bowls. Top with the bean sprouts, then ladle over the broth. Garnish with the spring onions and coriander. Serve with lime wedges to squeeze over.

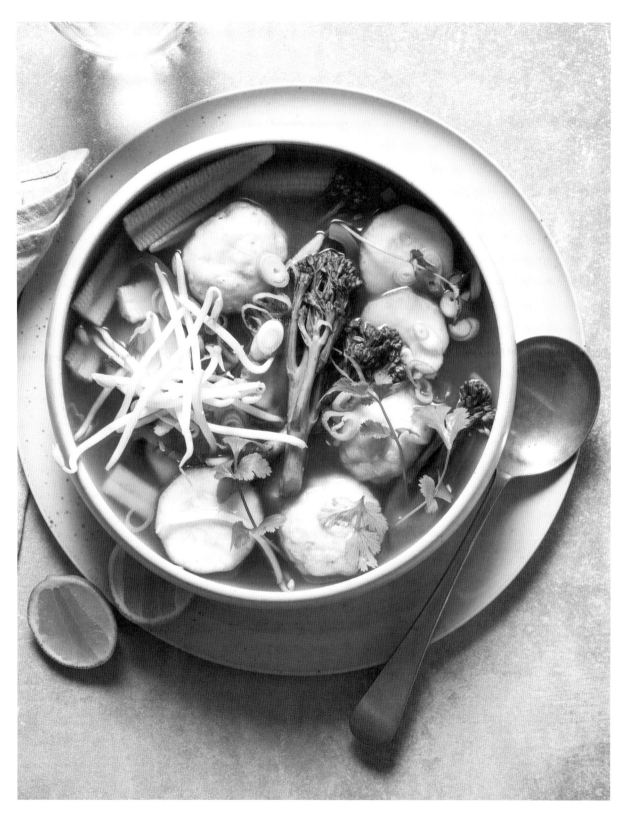

INFO PER SERVING: CALORIES 234   PROTEIN (G) 34   CARBS (G) 12.5   SUGAR (G) 8   FAT (G) 4
SATURATED FAT (G) 1.5   FIBRE (G) 5   SALT (G) 3.7

CHICKEN & SWEETCORN SOUP

2 tsp cornflour

pinch of sugar

pinch of salt

1 large skinless, boneless chicken breast, cut into very thin strips

1 tbsp soy sauce

1 litre chicken stock

5g root ginger, grated

2 garlic cloves, grated

3 spring onions, whites and greens separated and cut into rounds

a few coriander sprigs, finely chopped

400g frozen sweetcorn, defrosted

1 egg

sea salt and black pepper

To garnish

a few coriander leaves

sesame or chilli oil (optional)

This is a really proper chicken and sweetcorn soup. You could, of course, make it with ready-cooked chicken breast, but if you go the extra mile and do the velveting process as we suggest it's so much nicer. Velveting simply means marinating the chicken in a mixture of cornflour, sugar, salt and soy sauce, and it gives the meat a beautifully soft, tender texture. Try it and we're sure you'll agree. It elevates this takeaway favourite to something very special.

First prepare the chicken. Put the cornflour into a bowl and add pinches of sugar and salt. Toss the chicken in the seasoned cornflour, then pour over the soy sauce and mix thoroughly. Leave to marinate for at least an hour.

To make the soup, put the chicken stock in a large saucepan. Add the ginger, garlic, spring onion whites and coriander, then bring to the boil and simmer for 5 minutes. Taste and add salt and pepper as desired.

Put 300g of the sweetcorn in a food processor and purée until it's well broken down. Add this and the whole sweetcorn kernels to the soup and simmer for a further 5 minutes.

Drop the pieces of chicken into the soup, along with the spring onion greens and cook for a couple of minutes. Break the egg into a bowl and beat until smooth. Stir the soup in a fluid, circular motion, then slowly pour the egg into the pan from a height, continuing to stir as you do so. The egg will cook instantly and will have a thread-like consistency.

Remove the pan from the heat and ladle the soup into bowls. Garnish with the coriander and a few drops of oil, if using.

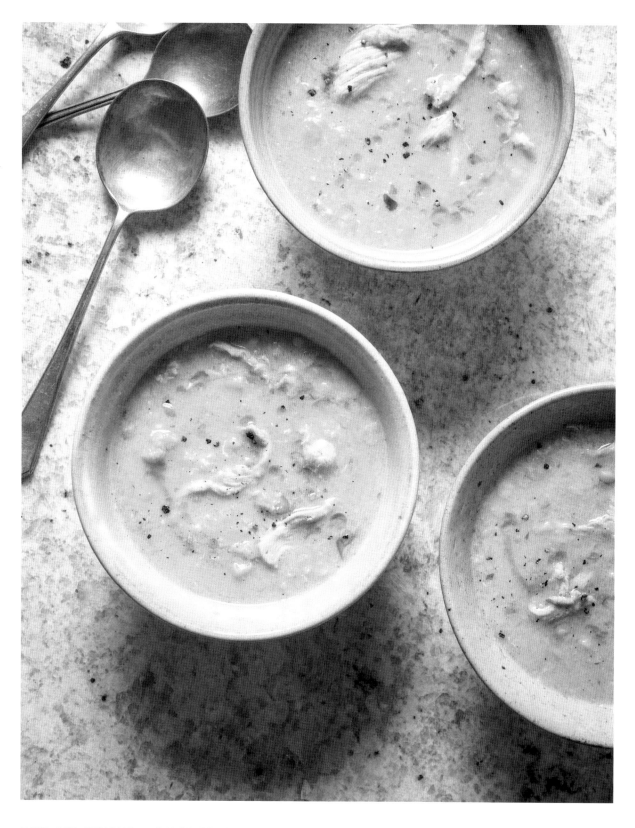

INFO PER SERVING: CALORIES 184   PROTEIN (G) 24   CARBS (G) 12   SUGAR (G) 4   FAT (G) 4
SATURATED FAT (G) 1   FIBRE (G) 2   SALT (G) 1.2

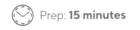
CELERIAC, APPLE & SMOKED MACKEREL SALAD

½ celeriac (about 200g), peeled

2 crisp eating apples, unpeeled and cored

juice of ½ lime

2 heads of white or red chicory

200g smoked mackerel fillets

1 tbsp capers

fronds from a small bunch of dill

small bunch of chives, snipped into short lengths

Dressing

50ml buttermilk or drinking kefir

1 tsp wholegrain mustard

½ tsp honey

2 tsp sherry vinegar

sea salt and black pepper

Celeriac is low in calories, so is an excellent choice when you're watching your weight. Its flavour marries perfectly with the sweetness of the apples and the smoky taste of the mackerel, and it's all brought together with the wonderful dressing. This is a salad with a perfect sweet/savoury balance.

First prepare the vegetables. Cut the celeriac into thin matchsticks, either with a sharp knife or by using a julienne tool. Cut the apples into very thin wedges, then toss the celeriac and the apples in the lime juice. Finely slice the outer leaves of the chicory and leave the small inner leaves whole.

Skin the mackerel fillets and pull the flesh into chunks.

Make the dressing by whisking the buttermilk or kefir with the mustard, honey and sherry vinegar. Season with salt and pepper.

Put the celeriac, apple, chicory, mackerel and capers into a bowl. Pour over the dressing and mix thoroughly. Stir in the dill and the snipped chives and serve.

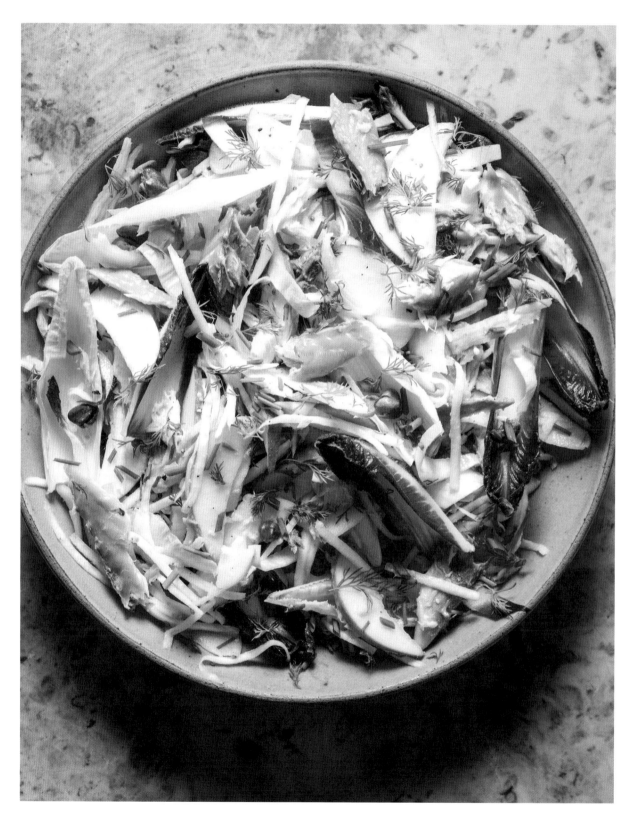

INFO PER SERVING: CALORIES 228   PROTEIN (G) 12.5   CARBS (G) 12.5   SUGAR (G) 10.5   FAT (G) 13
SATURATED FAT (G) 3   FIBRE (G) 4.5   SALT (G) 1.2

THAI TOFU SALAD

1 tsp vegetable oil

1 block of extra-firm tofu
(280g is about right), diced

½ Chinese lettuce/cabbage,
shredded

1 large carrot, cut into matchsticks

½ red pepper, cut into matchsticks

100g mangetout, trimmed and
shredded

100g baby corn, cut into rounds

50g bean sprouts

1 red chilli, finely chopped

leaves from a small bunch of
coriander

leaves from a small bunch of Thai
basil, roughly torn (optional)

Dressing

2 tbsp fish sauce

1 tbsp tamarind purée

1 tbsp palm sugar or light
soft brown sugar

juice of 1 lime

1 shallot, finely sliced

sea salt and black pepper

Peanut garnish

1 tsp vegetable oil

1 tsp palm sugar

2 tbsp lightly crushed peanuts

large pinch of chilli flakes or
powder

There are no calories in flavour and this salad is packed with great tastes. Tofu is a great flavour carrier and so it's just right for adding protein and texture to this satisfying vegan recipe. It makes a good light lunch and can be piled into a lunch box for a meal on the go. By the way, if you have tamarind concentrate rather than purée, just use a teaspoonful and dilute it.

First make the dressing. Whisk all the ingredients together until the sugar has completely dissolved. Taste and adjust the seasoning to get the flavour you like.

Next make the garnish. Heat the oil in a wok or a small frying pan. Add the remaining garnish ingredients along with a pinch of salt and then cook until the peanuts are well toasted. They should look glossy and browned. Tip them on to some kitchen paper to drain – they should be crisp and sticky by the time they have cooled.

For the tofu, heat the oil in a wok or frying pan. When the oil is smoking, add the tofu and stir-fry until it is lightly browned. Remove the tofu from the wok and toss it in a tablespoon of the dressing.

Put the prepared vegetables and the bean sprouts in a large bowl or platter and toss them lightly to combine. Drizzle over the remaining dressing, top with the tofu and sprinkle with the chilli, herbs and the peanut garnish.

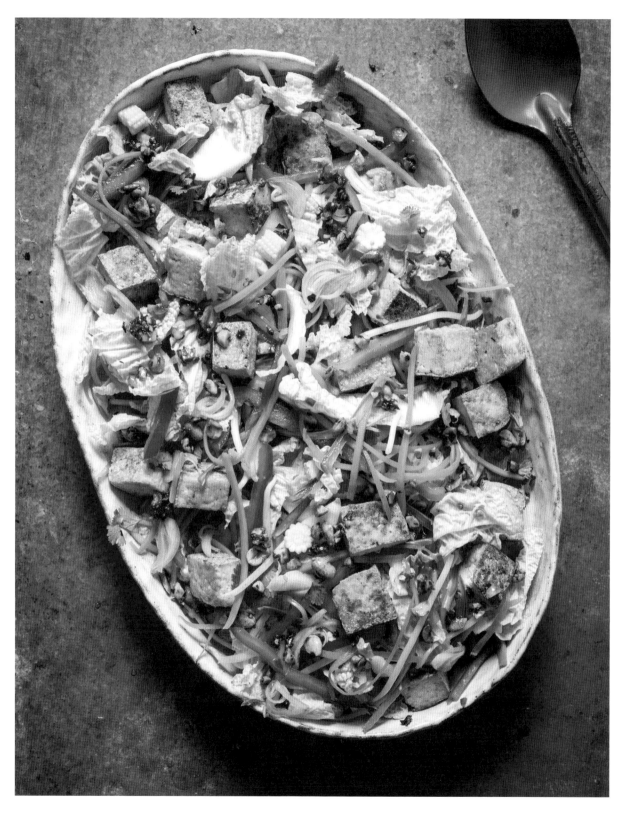

INFO PER SERVING: CALORIES 231   PROTEIN (G) 14.5   CARBS (G) 15.5   SUGAR (G) 13   FAT (G) 11
SATURATED FAT (G) 2   FIBRE (G) 6   SALT (G) 1.5

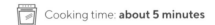
ZESTY SQUID & WHITE BEAN SALAD

juice and zest of 1 lime

1 tsp smoked chilli paste or sauce
(chipotle is good)

1 tsp olive oil

1 tsp sherry or cider vinegar

1 garlic clove, crushed

pinch of sugar

300g squid, cleaned and cut
into rings

sea salt and black pepper

Salad

200g cherry tomatoes

150g runner or flat beans,
shredded

400g can of cannellini or butter
beans, drained

1 small courgette, very finely sliced
into rounds

2 spring onions, very finely sliced
into rounds

100g salad leaves

2 mild red chillies, finely sliced

small bunch of coriander, finely
chopped

leaves from a few mint sprigs, torn

a few basil leaves, torn

Squid is available in supermarkets now and comes all cleaned and prepped so there are no messy bits to worry about. This way of cooking it is even quicker than grilling and, as the squid benefits from sitting in the marinade, it's a good prepare-ahead dish. It gives you a taste of Mediterranean summer at any time of year.

First prepare the marinade for the squid. Put the lime juice and zest in a bowl with the chilli paste or sauce, olive oil, vinegar and garlic. Add salt, pepper, a generous pinch of sugar and a tablespoon of water and mix thoroughly.

Bring a large saucepan of water to the boil. Add plenty of salt and drop in the squid. Cook until you can see the squid has turned opaque – this will take 30 seconds to 1 minute. Drain immediately, then drop the squid into the marinade mixture and toss well. Cover the bowl and leave the squid to marinate for at least half an hour, preferably an hour.

Roughly chop the cherry tomatoes, then strain them over a bowl. Add any strained juices to the squid and mix well. Add the runner or flat beans to a pan of boiling water and cook for a few minutes, then drain and rinse under cold water.

Put both types of beans, the cherry tomatoes, courgette, spring onions and salad leaves in a salad bowl or serving dish and add the squid and all the marinade. Mix thoroughly, then add the chillies and herbs. Toss very gently and serve at room temperature.

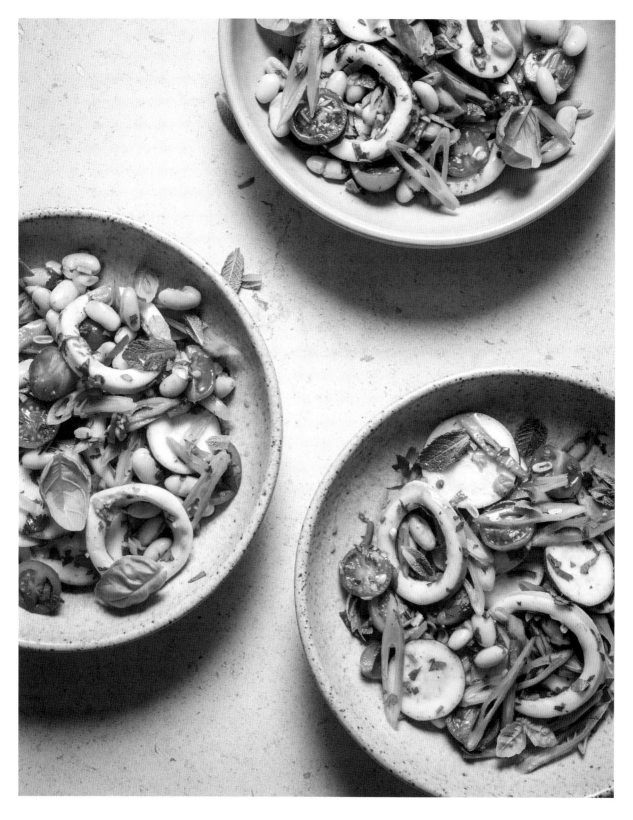

INFO PER SERVING: CALORIES 171   PROTEIN (G) 18   CARBS (G) 15   SUGAR (G) 5   FAT (G) 3
SATURATED FAT (G) 0.5   FIBRE (G) 7   SALT (G) 0.2

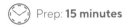

SERRANO HAM SALAD

2 oranges

100g rocket or 1 cos lettuce, shredded

1 small red onion, sliced into crescents

2 roast peppers from a jar, cut into strips

100g radishes, sliced into rounds

6 slices of Serrano ham, pulled into strips

leaves from a fresh oregano sprig

leaves from a couple of parsley sprigs

25g hazelnuts, lightly crushed

Dressing

2 tsp olive oil or hazelnut oil

1 tsp sherry vinegar

sea salt and black pepper

Quick, fresh and delicious, this makes a nice light lunch that's as satisfying to the eye as it is to the palate. With the sharpness of the chicory, sweetness of the orange and savoury hit of ham, its flavours are perfectly balanced. The crushed hazelnuts and crisp radishes add some crunch. Rocket or lettuce both work well but so do bitter leaves, such as chicory. We use roast peppers from a jar for speed and suggest you do the same. If you do have some hazelnut oil in your cupboard this is a great use for it, as it will echo the flavour of the nuts in the salad.

Peel the oranges carefully, removing all the white pith, and slice them into thin rounds. Take the discarded peel and squeeze any juice into a bowl. To make the dressing, add the oil and vinegar to the bowl with the juice, season with salt and pepper, then whisk to combine.

Place the rocket or lettuce, onion, peppers, radishes, orange slices and ham on a serving dish and toss gently. Sprinkle over the herbs and crushed hazelnuts, then drizzle the dressing over the salad and serve right away.

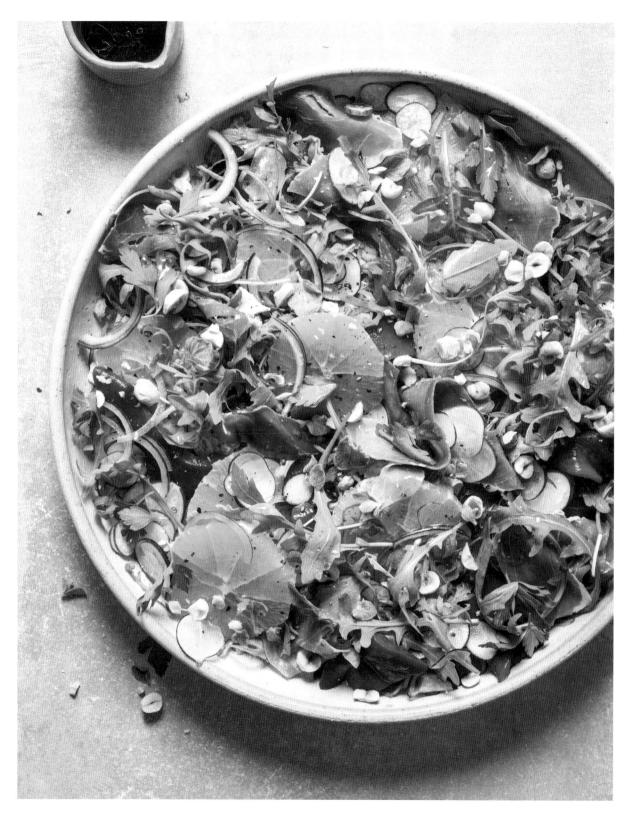

INFO PER SERVING: CALORIES 151   PROTEIN (G) 10   CARBS (G) 8   SUGAR (G) 7.5   FAT (G) 8
SATURATED FAT (G) 1.5   FIBRE (G) 2.5   SALT (G) 1.4

JACKFRUIT & COCONUT CURRY

1 tsp coconut oil
12 curry leaves
3 green chillies, left whole,
    slit lengthways
1 tsp mustard seeds
2 medium onions, finely sliced
15g root ginger, finely chopped
3 garlic cloves, finely chopped
1 tbsp mild curry powder
300g pumpkin or squash, diced
400g can of jackfruit, drained
400g reduced-fat coconut milk
1 tbsp tamarind purée
    (1 tsp if using concentrate)
150g mangetout or sugar
    snap peas
sea salt and black pepper

To serve
small bunch of coriander,
    roughly chopped
squeeze of lime juice

Often called a superfood, jackfruit is low in calories and has an uncanny similarity to pulled pork! It's available in cans in the supermarkets and is ideal for tasty vegan dishes, like this curry, as it has a satisfying meaty texture and marries well with spicy flavours. It contains no saturated fat or cholesterol so is a great healthy choice.

Heat the coconut oil in a flameproof casserole dish or a saucepan. Add the curry leaves, chillies and mustard seeds. When they start crackling, add the onions. Stir and add a splash of water, then cover the pan and leave to cook over a medium heat for about 10 minutes, stirring regularly.

Add the ginger and garlic and stir for a couple of minutes, then stir in the curry powder. Add the pumpkin or squash and the jackfruit, then stir so it's all well coated with the spices. Pour in the coconut milk and about 100ml of water, then add the tamarind purée and season with salt and pepper.

Bring to the boil, then turn the heat down and simmer for about 15 minutes. Add the mangetout or sugar snap peas and continue to simmer until the vegetables are completely tender. Check the seasoning and add the coriander and a squeeze of lime juice.

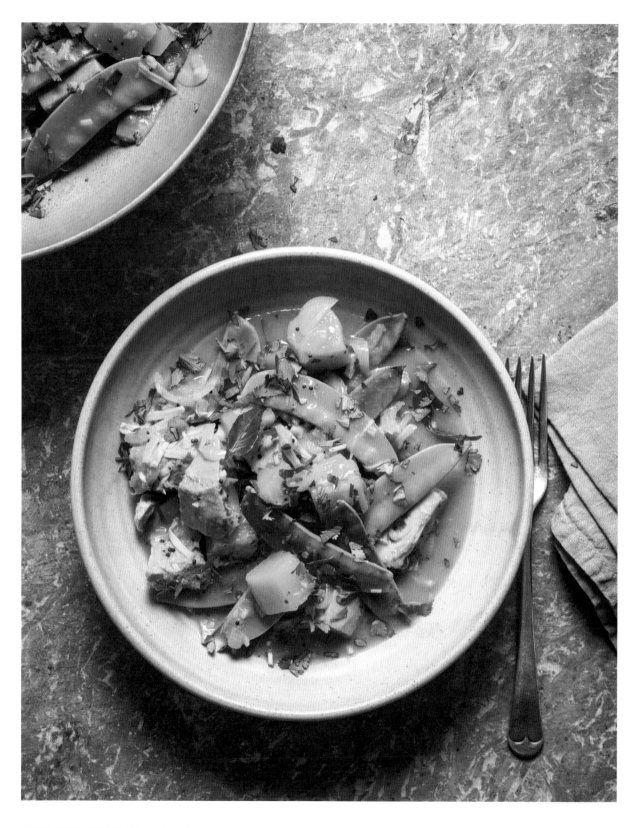

INFO PER SERVING: CALORIES 173   PROTEIN (G) 4   CARBS (G) 15   SUGAR (G) 9   FAT (G) 9
SATURATED FAT (G) 7   FIBRE (G) 6   SALT (G) 0.1

EPIC BRAISED LENTILS

1 tbsp olive oil
1 large onion, finely chopped
1 large carrot, finely diced
2 celery sticks, finely chopped
3 garlic cloves, finely chopped
250g puy lentils
½ tsp fennel seeds
1 tsp smoked chilli flakes
     or paprika
1 strip of pared lemon zest
1 bay leaf
leaves from a sprig of oregano,
     finely chopped
200ml red or white wine
600ml vegetable or chicken stock
     or water
sea salt and black pepper

To serve
leaves from a few sprigs of parsley,
     finely chopped

This is our go-to way of cooking lentils and we hope it becomes yours too. Lentils are a good source of protein and not too high in calories, so are just the thing when you want something nourishing which won't bust the diet. Enjoy this on its own for supper or as a side dish with some salmon or grilled chicken – don't forget to add calories for any extras though, if you're counting .

Heat the olive oil in a large saucepan. Add the vegetables and sauté them over a high heat until they're starting to soften and brown around the edges. Add the garlic and cook for another couple of minutes, then stir in the lentils, fennel seeds, chilli flakes or paprika, lemon zest and herbs. Season with salt and pepper – lentils need plenty of salt, so don't stint.

Pour in the wine and bring to the boil. Continue to boil for 2 minutes, then add the stock or water. Bring back to the boil, then turn the heat down to somewhere between a boil and a simmer and cover the pan. Cook for 35–40 minutes until the vegetables and lentils are tender. Check regularly, giving everything a quick stir to make sure the lentils aren't sticking, and add a splash more liquid towards the end if the mixture is getting too dry.

Remove the lemon zest and serve sprinkled with parsley.

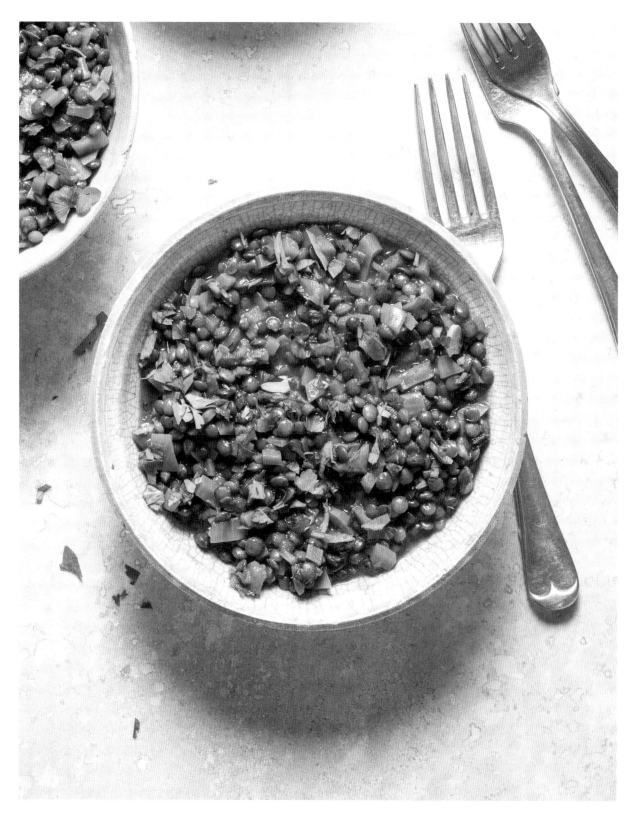

INFO PER SERVING: CALORIES 207   PROTEIN (G) 11.5   CARBS (G) 18   SUGAR (G) 6   FAT (G) 4
SATURATED FAT (G) 0.8   FIBRE (G) 6.5   SALT (G) TRACE

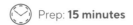
LOUISIANA-STYLE VEGETABLE KEBABS

16 okra, trimmed

16 closed-cup mushrooms

1 corn on the cob, cut into 8 pieces

1 red pepper, cut into chunks

1 green pepper, cut into chunks

4 spring onions, cut into
　3cm rounds

Seasoning

½ tsp garlic powder

½ tsp onion powder

½ tsp dried thyme

½ tsp cumin

½ tsp sweet smoked paprika

dash of Tabasco or similar
　hot sauce

1 tbsp olive oil

squeeze of lemon juice

sea salt and black pepper

To serve

lemon wedges

hot sauce

Buttermilk dressing (optional)

150ml buttermilk

75g crème fraiche

2 tsp cider vinegar

½ tsp garlic powder

pinch of sugar

a few basil leaves, finely chopped

a few chives, finely chopped

Here's a recipe inspired by our days filming down on the Mississippi Delta. The best way to get the tasty coating on these veggie kebabs is to get your hands in there and get messy – much more effective than brushing. These kebabs are great cooked on a barbecue or grill and can be served with our delicious buttermilk dressing or just with hot sauce and lemon juice.

Preheat a grill to its highest setting or prepare a barbecue. You will need 8 skewers and if using bamboo skewers, soak them in warm water for half an hour first.

Mix all the seasoning ingredients together in a large bowl with some salt and pepper and a tablespoon of water. Add all the vegetables and mix with your hands until they are very well coated in the seasoning.

Thread the vegetables on to the skewers, making sure each one has at least 2 pieces of okra, 2 mushrooms and a piece of corn. Arrange the skewers on a rack for the grill or on the barbecue. Cook for 4–5 minutes on each side until the veg are slightly charred and softened.

To make the dressing, if using, mix everything together and season with salt and pepper. Serve with the kebabs.

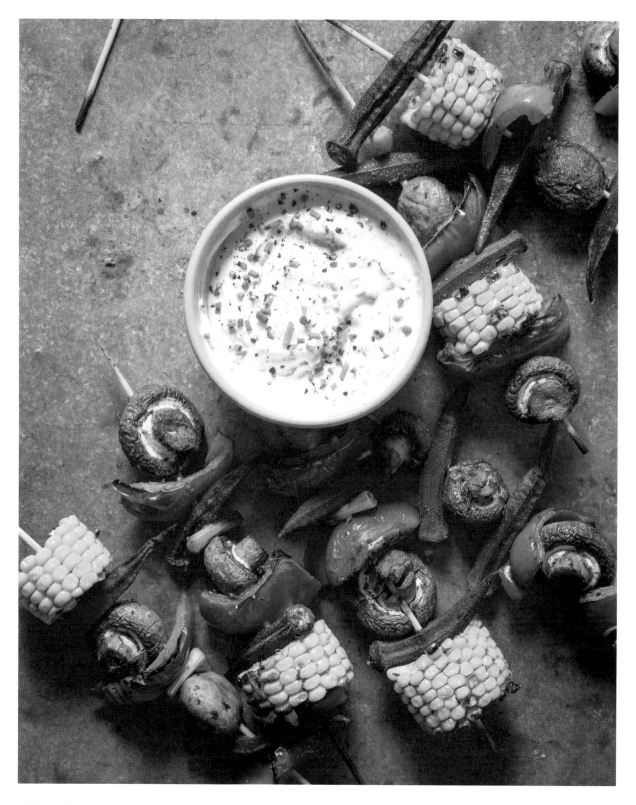

INFO PER SERVING WITHOUT DRESSING/WITH DRESSING: CALORIES 84/170   PROTEIN (G) 3/5
CARBS (G) 6.5/9   SUGAR (G) 5/7   FAT (G) 4/7   SATURATED FAT (G) 0.5/6   FIBRE (G) 5/5
SALT (G) TRACE/TRACE

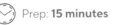

STUFFED VEGETABLES

2 large peppers or 4 small peppers
or 4 beefsteak tomatoes (or
similar) or 4 round courgettes
sea salt and black pepper

Stuffing
2 tsp olive oil
2 baby leeks or 4 spring onions,
cut into rounds
100g asparagus tips, cut into
rounds
1 small courgette (about 100g),
diced
150g cooked quinoa (50g
uncooked)
zest and juice of ½ lime
leaves from small bunches of mint
and parsley, finely chopped
a few basil leaves, shredded
leaves from a large tarragon sprig,
finely chopped
50g Cheddar or hard goat's
cheese, grated

For us, stuffed vegetables have never been out of fashion. In our new version, the stuffing is made of lots of veg and some quinoa, so is lighter than the usual rice mix and very tasty indeed. Whether you opt for peppers, tomatoes or courgettes, we reckon this is the way to go.

Preheat the oven to 200°C/Fan 180°C/Gas 6. If using large peppers, cut them in half lengthways through the core and remove any seeds and white bits from the insides. If using 4 small peppers, tomatoes or courgettes, cut off the tops and remove the insides. Reserve the flesh of the tomatoes or courgettes for use in another recipe.

If using peppers or courgettes, put them in an ovenproof dish and season with salt and pepper. Roast in the oven for 15 minutes. Tomatoes will be fine just cooked with the stuffing.

To make the filling, heat a teaspoon of the oil in a frying pan. Add the leeks or spring onions, asparagus tips and courgette and fry briskly over a high heat for a few minutes. The aim is to give them a little colour and get them to the firm side of al dente. Put them in a bowl with the quinoa, lime zest and juice and the herbs. Season with salt and pepper.

Reserve 4 teaspoonfuls of the cheese and stir the rest into the stuffing mixture. Divide the mixture between the peppers, tomatoes or courgettes – each one should take just over 100g. Sprinkle with the reserved cheese. Mix the remaining oil with a half teaspoon of water and use this to brush over the cut surface of the vegetables and the top of the stuffing.

Roast in the oven for about 20 minutes, until the vegetables have softened and are browning around the edges. Nice with a salad.

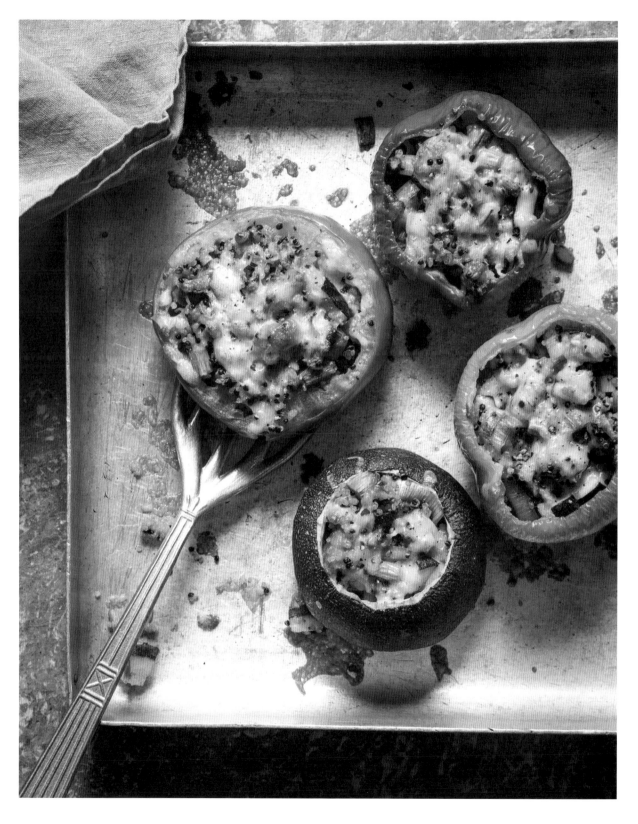

INFO PER SERVING: CALORIES 158   PROTEIN (G) 8   CARBS (G) 13   SUGAR (G) 6.5   FAT (G) 7
SATURATED FAT (G) 3   FIBRE (G) 5.5   SALT (G) TRACE

LEMON-CRUSTED ROAST COD

4 pieces of cod loin or similar
  (about 150g each)

Crust
2 tbsp capers
2 tbsp green olives, pitted
zest of 1 lemon
juice of ½ lemon
1 tbsp Dijon mustard
leaves from 2 basil sprigs,
  finely chopped
leaves from 4 parsley sprigs,
  finely chopped
sea salt and black pepper

Beans
1 tsp olive oil
300g runner or stringless beans,
  finely shredded
3 garlic cloves, finely chopped

In this recipe, a nice bit of cod is livened up with a really zesty, tasty coat. It's so simple to do and makes a great quick supper with some green beans and white bean mash if you fancy (see page 168 for the mash). The bean method also works well with thinly sliced courgettes, shredded chard or kale.

Preheat the oven to 200°C/Fan 180°C/Gas 6. Line a baking tray with baking parchment.

For the crust, put all the ingredients in a small food processor with plenty of black pepper, then pulse until you have a rough paste. Season the fish fillets and spread each one with the paste. Place them on the baking tray and bake in the oven for about 15 minutes.

While the fish is cooking, cook the beans. Heat the olive oil in a pan and add the beans. Stir to coat them with the oil and add the garlic. Season with salt and pepper, add a splash of water and cover the pan. Braise the beans gently until tender, shaking the pan regularly.

Serve the fish with the green beans and some white bean mash (see page 168).

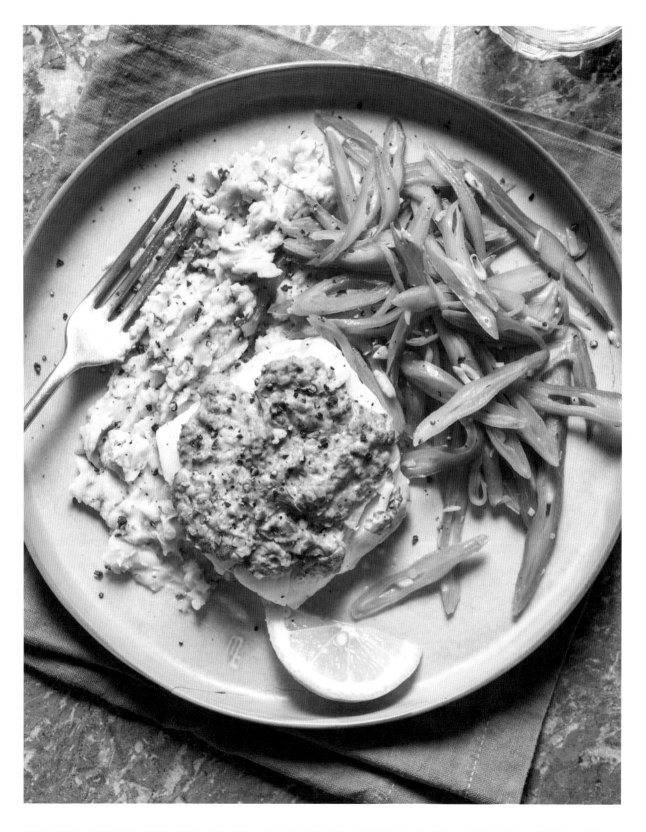

INFO PER SERVING (COD AND BEANS): CALORIES 162 PROTEIN (G) 28 CARBS (G) 3 SUGAR (G) 2.5 FAT (G) 3.5 SATURATED FAT (G) O.5 FIBRE (G) 2.5 SALT (G) 1

Serves: **4** Prep: **15 minutes** + chilling Cooking time: **about 45 minutes**

COD & HAM CROQUETTES

300g potatoes, unpeeled
 and cut into chunks
200g cod fillet, skinned
milk, to cover
1 bay leaf
a few black peppercorns, crushed
4 slices of Serrano ham, finely
 chopped
sea salt and black pepper

Coating
15g plain flour
1 egg, beaten
50g dried breadcrumbs
 (such as panko)

Croquettes are usually deep-fried but we've found that you can bake them in the oven – they're still delicious and lower in fat! You don't need a lot of coating so the calorie count is reasonable. The key to success is making sure the potatoes and the cod are really dry before making the mixture. If it's too wet, the croquettes will steam and might burst in the oven. And we wouldn't want that to happen to our tasty little morsels.

Put the potatoes in a steamer basket set over a pan of simmering water and season with salt. Cover and steam until the potatoes are tender. Tip them into a bowl, cover with a tea towel and leave to absorb excess moisture for 10 minutes. Remove the skins and mash.

While the potatoes are cooking, put the cod in a small saucepan with just enough milk to cover. Add the bay leaf and peppercorns. Bring to the boil, then cover the pan and remove it from the heat. Leave until cool, then remove the fish from the milk, drain thoroughly, then flake the flesh on to kitchen paper.

Mix the potato and fish together with the chopped ham and plenty of seasoning. Chill until the mixture is firm – at least an hour. Preheat the oven to 200°C/Fan 180°C/Gas 6 and line a baking tray with some baking parchment.

Divide the mixture into 12 and shape into croquettes or little balls. Put the flour, egg and half the breadcrumbs in separate shallow bowls. Dip each croquette into the flour, pat off any excess, then dip into the egg followed by the breadcrumbs. Continue until all the croquettes are nicely coated, topping up the breadcrumbs halfway through.

Place the croquettes on a baking tray and bake for 12–15 minutes until golden brown and piping hot. Keep a close eye on them after 12 minutes – they can burst if over cooked. Serve hot, with a tomato and red onion salad (see page 170).

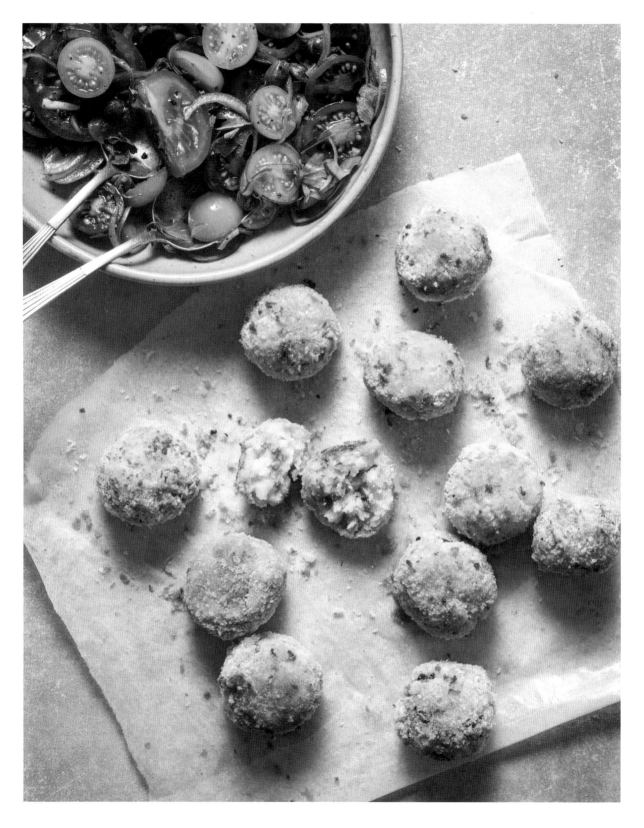

INFO PER SERVING: CALORIES 214   PROTEIN (G) 18   CARBS (G) 26   SUGAR (G) 1.5   FAT (G) 3.5
SATURATED FAT (G) 1   FIBRE (G) 1.5   SALT (G) 1

CHICKEN & SPINACH CURRY

1 large onion, roughly chopped

4 garlic cloves, roughly chopped

15g root ginger, peeled and roughly chopped

1 tsp coconut oil, ghee or vegetable oil

1 tsp mustard seeds

1 tsp cumin seeds

1 tbsp curry powder

1 tbsp tomato purée

4 skinless chicken thigh fillets, diced

200ml chicken stock or water

500g frozen chopped spinach, defrosted

small bunch of coriander, finely chopped

100g plain yoghurt

juice of ½ lemon

sea salt and black pepper

Chicken is lower in calories than lamb and makes a delicious saag curry that's so easy to do. As we all know, spinach is rich in iron which is an important nutrient, but we need some vitamin C as well to help us absorb it. So here's a top tip – add a touch of fresh lemon juice to the curry right at the end before serving.

Put the onion, garlic cloves and ginger into a food processor and whizz to form a purée.

Heat the oil in a large saucepan or a flameproof casserole dish. Add the mustard and cumin seeds, then fry them until they pop. Stir in the curry powder for a minute, then add the onion purée and continue to fry for a few minutes until the mixture is very aromatic and reduced.

Stir in the tomato purée and continue to cook, stirring constantly until everything is well combined and the tomato purée has lost its raw edge. Add the diced chicken and stir until it's all well coated in the spicy purée.

Pour in the stock or water and stir to make sure the base of the pan is thoroughly deglazed, then stir in the spinach and most of the coriander. Season with salt and pepper. Bring to the boil, then turn the heat down and simmer for 15 minutes, until the chicken is completely cooked through and tender, and the sauce has reduced a little.

Stir in the yoghurt and leave to simmer for a couple of minutes, being careful not to let the mixture boil. Add the lemon juice before serving and garnish with the reserved coriander.

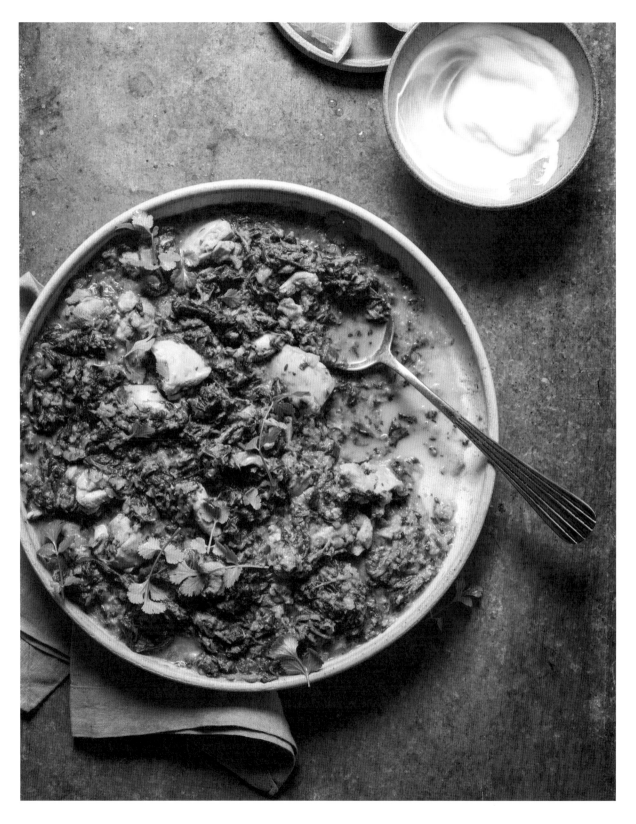

INFO PER SERVING: CALORIES 200   PROTEIN (G) 24   CARBS (G) 9   SUGAR (G) 7   FAT (G) 6
SATURATED FAT (G) 2   FIBRE (G) 6   SALT (G) 0.8

CORONATION CHICKEN COLESLAW

1 small white or pointed green
  cabbage (about 300g),
  shredded
150g celeriac, cut into matchsticks
1 large carrot, cut into matchsticks
4 spring onions, finely sliced
1 apple (unpeeled), cored and
  grated
25g raisins, soaked in warm water
2 cooked skinless, boneless
  chicken breasts, shredded
squeeze of lemon or lime juice
small bunch of coriander, finely
  chopped
sea salt and black pepper

Sauce
150g yoghurt
zest and juice of ½ lime
1 tsp mild curry powder
½ tsp garlic powder
½ tsp chilli powder or flakes
1 tbsp mango chutney
½ tsp each nigella and mustard
  seeds

To serve
leaves from 3 little gem lettuces

A fab twist on a great old favourite – we reckon this would be great with leftover turkey on Boxing Day, too. It's good just on its own but you might like to take things up a notch and serve it on little lettuce leaf boats.

Put the cabbage, celeriac, carrot, spring onions and apple into a colander. Sprinkle with a teaspoon of salt and leave for half an hour. This will help draw out some of the liquid from the vegetables and give you a crisper coleslaw.

Squeeze the vegetables gently and transfer them to a bowl. Drain the raisins. Sprinkle the chicken with salt and pepper and squeeze over the lemon or lime juice. Toss together, then add the chicken to the vegetables along with the raisins and coriander.

Mix all the sauce ingredients together and season. Taste and adjust the amount of chilli, if you need to, then pour the sauce over the vegetables and chicken. Mix thoroughly (the easiest, if messiest, way is to use your hands). Serve as is in bowls, or spoon into lettuce leaves.

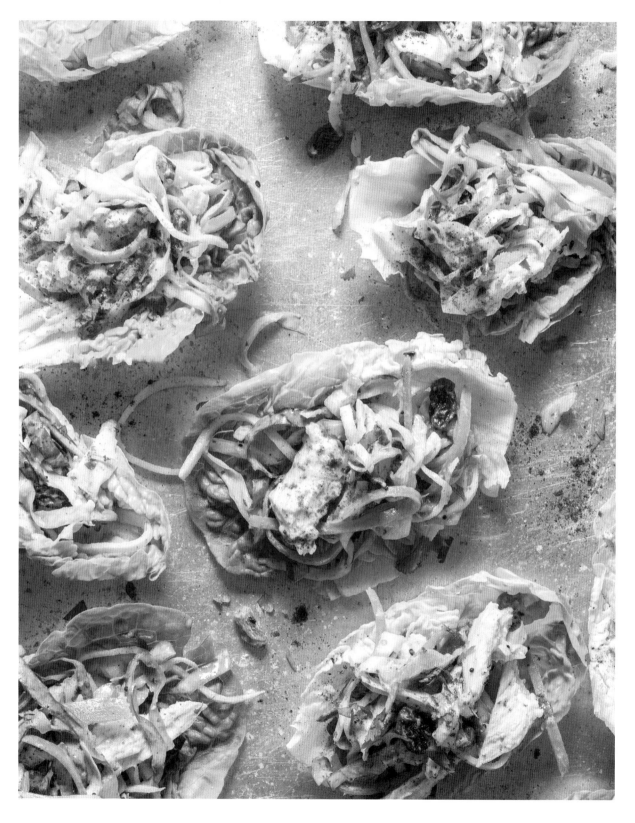

INFO PER SERVING: CALORIES 245   PROTEIN (G) 27.5   CARBS (G) 19   SUGAR (G) 18   FAT (G) 5
SATURATED FAT (G) 1.5   FIBRE (G) 7   SALT (G) TRACE

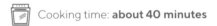
MOROCCAN CHICKEN

2 tsp olive oil
1 onion, finely chopped
3 garlic cloves, finely chopped
1 tsp ground ginger
½ tsp cinnamon
¼ tsp ground allspice
¼ tsp ground cloves
¼– ½ tsp cayenne (to taste)
4 skinless chicken thigh fillets,
    trimmed and cut in half
250ml chicken stock
pinch of saffron, soaked in warm
    water
1 preserved lemon, finely chopped
4 artichoke hearts, halved
200g green beans, trimmed
12 green olives, pitted
sea salt and black pepper

To garnish
peel from 1 preserved lemon,
    finely chopped
leaves from a few mint sprigs,
    finely chopped
leaves from a few parsley sprigs,
    finely chopped

A fabulously spicy, warming dish, this is a variation on a Moroccan tagine. If you prefer, you could use 2 teaspoons of ras-el-hanout instead of the individual spices. Great served with a low-calorie cauliflower pilaf (see page 172) or with couscous if you like.

Heat the oil in a saucepan or a flameproof casserole dish. Add the onion and sauté until it starts to soften. Add the garlic and sauté for a minute, then stir in the spices. Add the chicken pieces and turn them over to coat them in the spices.

Pour in the stock and saffron, then sprinkle in the preserved lemon and season with salt and pepper. Tuck in the artichoke hearts and put the green beans on top – they will steam as the chicken cooks. Sprinkle over the olives. Bring to the boil, then cover and turn the heat down to a simmer. Leave to cook for about half an hour, until the chicken and beans are tender.

For the garnish, mix the preserved lemon peel and herbs together and sprinkle over the dish before serving.

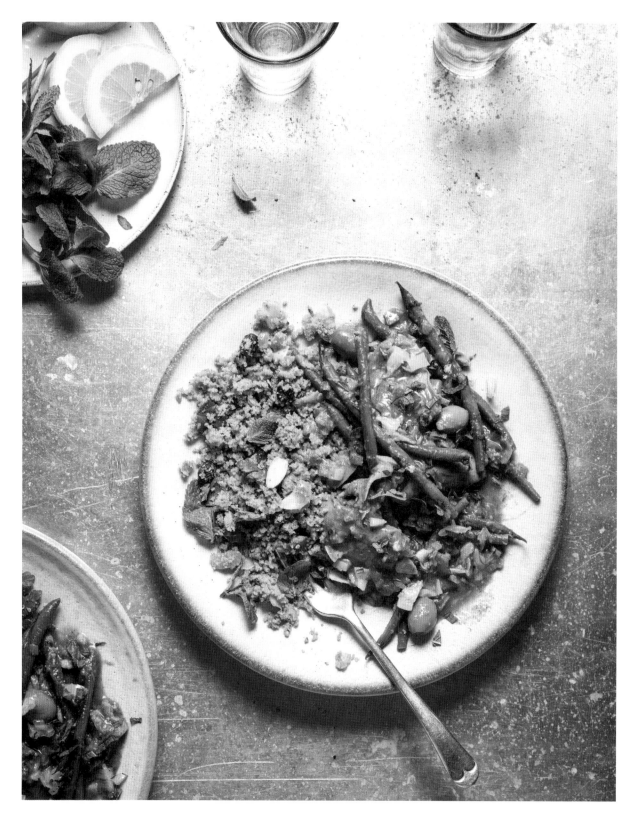

INFO PER SERVING (NOT INCLUDING PILAF):   CALORIES 167   PROTEIN (G) 20   CARBS (G) 8
SUGAR (G) 7   FAT (G) 5   SATURATED FAT (G) 1   FIBRE (G) 5   SALT (G) 1.3

SOME
TO SN
ON

THING
ACK

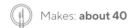 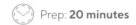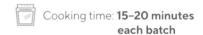
SEEDED CRACKERS

250g wholemeal flour, any sort, plus extra for dusting
½ tsp baking powder
½ tsp salt
100g mixed seeds
30ml olive oil
1 tsp honey
25g Parmesan or similar, grated (optional)

A tasty little number, these are spot on for scooping up the yummy dips you'll find on pages 86–89 and they're dead easy to make. Bake the whole lot in a couple of batches or stash some of the dough away in the freezer to bake another time. You can make them bigger if you like and add any other flavours you fancy. We recommend using at least 100g of wholemeal rye flour for the best flavour, and the seeds can be any combo of milled flax, chia, sesame, pumpkin and sunflower.

Preheat the oven to 200°C/Fan 180°C/Gas 6 and line 2 baking trays with baking parchment.

Put the flour, baking powder, salt and mixed seeds into a bowl and drizzle in the olive oil and honey. Gradually mix in up to 100ml of water, until you have a slightly sticky dough. Turn out on to a floured work surface and knead for a few minutes until the dough is firm but no longer tacky.

Divide the dough into 4 pieces. Roll out a piece as thinly as you can – it should be the depth of the largest type of seed you have used. If you have a meat cleaver, bash the dough all over with the dimpled side of the cleaver. Alternatively, prick the dough all over with a fork. Sprinkle with a quarter of the cheese, if using, and gently press the cheese into the dough.

Cut the dough into rectangles or rounds and place them on one of the baking trays. Repeat with the second piece of dough. Bake the crackers in the oven for 15–20 minutes until they are crisp and golden brown – make sure they are completely hard and dry. Remove from the oven. Repeat with the remaining pieces of dough.

These will keep in an airtight tin for at least a week.

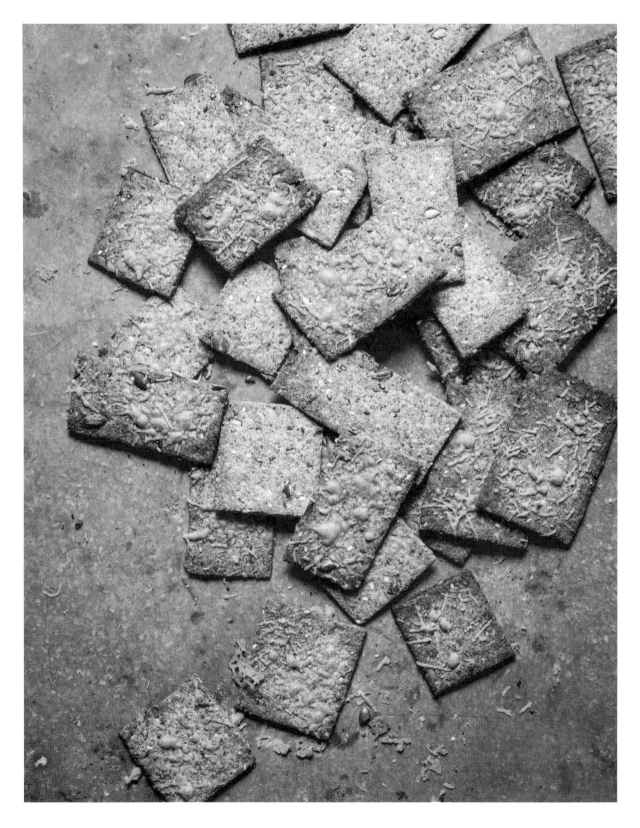

INFO PER CRACKER/WITH PARMESAN: CALORIES 37/40   PROTEIN (G) 1/1.5   CARBS (G) 5/5

SUGAR (G) 0.5/0.5 FAT (G) 1/1.5 SATURATED FAT (G) 0.3/0.5 FIBRE (G) 1/1 SALT (G)   TRACE/0.8

KIMCHI OMELETTE BAGUETTE

50g cabbage (white or green pointed), very finely shredded

1 medium carrot, coarsely grated or cut into matchsticks

1 spring onion, finely chopped

3 tbsp kimchi (see p.176 or shop-bought), drained and finely chopped

4 eggs

2 tsp butter

25g Cheddar, grated

sea salt and black pepper

To serve

2 x 15cm lengths of baguette (or similar)

a few drops of sesame oil

a few slices of cucumber

a few coriander sprigs

chilli sauce, chilli jam or ketchup

We reckon the best bit about a baguette is the crust – and of course, the doughy inside is where the calories are. So, the answer is to remove the soft inside and then you have a lovely crunchy sandwich to fill with this tasty kimchi omelette or whatever else you choose. Magic, eh?

First prepare the pieces of baguette. Split them in half lengthways and remove most of the soft bread inside. You can dry this out and use it for breadcrumbs – no need for any waste.

Divide the cabbage, carrot, chopped spring onion and kimchi between 2 bowls. Beat 2 of the eggs and add to one of the bowls, then beat the remaining eggs and add to the other bowl. Mix thoroughly and season with salt and pepper.

Heat a teaspoon of butter in an omelette pan. When it has melted, add the contents of one the bowls, swirling the mixture around to coat the base of the pan, then leave to cook until the underside is browned. Carefully flip the omelette over to cook the other side. Sprinkle over half the cheese, so it starts to melt on the top side. Now fold the omelette over, so the cheese is in the centre. Repeat the process with the second batch of ingredients.

Pile the omelettes into the baguettes and dress with a few drops of sesame oil, the cucumber and coriander, followed by the chilli condiment or ketchup of your choice.

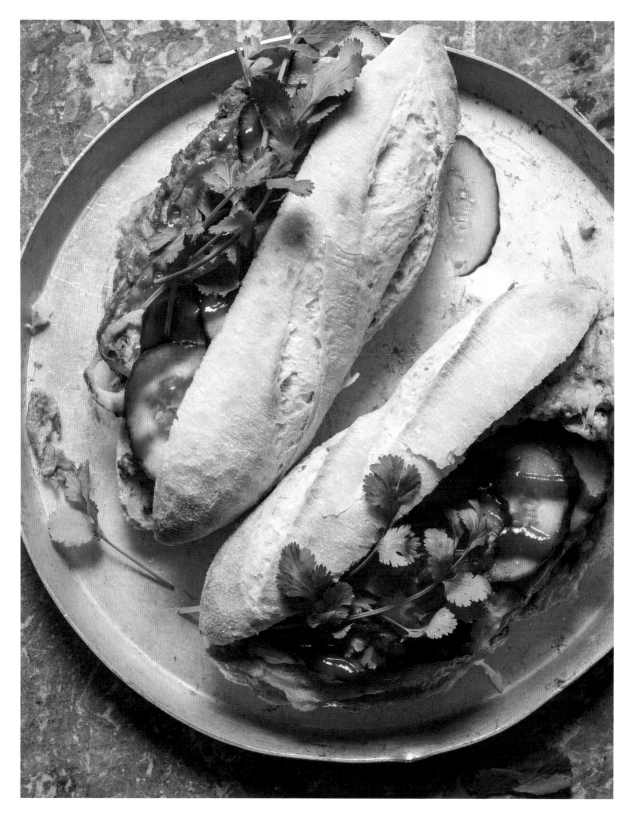

INFO PER SERVING: CALORIES 480   PROTEIN (G) 25   CARBS (G) 60   SUGAR (G) 8   FAT (G) 14
SATURATED FAT (G) 3.5   FIBRE (G) 6.5   SALT (G) 1.6

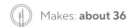
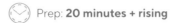
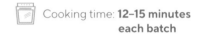
MARMITE BREADSTICKS

300g strong white bread flour,
    plus extra for dusting
5g fast-action dried yeast
1 tbsp olive oil
200ml tepid water
1 tsp Marmite
1 tsp honey

Glaze
1 tbsp Marmite
1 tbsp olive oil
1 tbsp hot water

People who love Marmite can't get enough of it and its deeply savoury flavour makes a great addition to these super-charged Twiglets. We warn you – you won't be able to stop eating them. They make a nice snack on their own or with one of the dips on pages 86–89. Top tip: be sure to combine the oil and Marmite well before adding water, otherwise it's hard to get it to emulsify.

First make the dough. Put the flour in a bowl with the yeast and drizzle in the oil. Measure the water into a jug and whisk in the Marmite and honey. Gradually add the Marmite water to the flour until you have a slightly sticky dough.

Dust your work surface with flour and turn out the dough. Knead until it is soft and very elastic, then try the windowpane test. To do this, break off a small piece of dough and stretch it out until it's so thin you can almost see through it. If you can do this, the gluten has developed enough and the dough is ready, but if the dough breaks, knead it for longer. If you prefer, knead the dough in a stand mixer.

Put the dough back in the bowl and cover with a damp cloth. Leave to rise for at least an hour until doubled in size.

When the dough has almost finished proving, line 2 baking trays with baking parchment. To make the glaze, mix the Marmite with the olive oil until completely combined, then whisk in the hot water. Preheat the oven to 220°C/Fan 200°C/Gas 7.

Knock back the dough to deflate it, then turn it out again on to the work surface. Roll the dough as thinly as possible into a large rectangle, then cut it into about 36 thin strips – this is easiest with a pizza wheel. Take each strip and twist it, then arrange half of the strips on the baking trays – it's best to cook them in 2 batches.

Brush the breadsticks with the Marmite glaze, then place in the preheated oven. Bake for 12–15 minutes until a rich brown. Remove from the oven and allow the trays to cool completely before repeating with the remaining breadsticks. Store in an airtight tin.

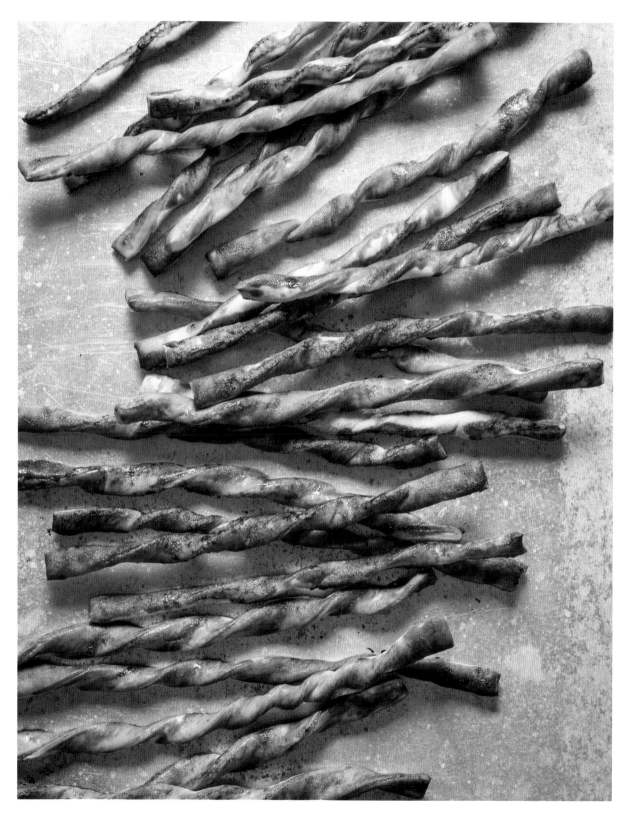

INFO PER STICK: CALORIES 38   PROTEIN (G) 1   CARBS (G) 6.5   SUGAR (G) 0.5   FAT (G) 0.7
SATURATED FAT (G) 0.1   FIBRE (G) 0.3   SALT (G) 0.06

SMASHING SANDWICHES

Salmon & cottage cheese

213g can of salmon or tuna
150g cottage cheese
2 tbsp roughly chopped capers
1 tbsp tarragon or Dijon mustard
1 large tarragon sprig, finely
    chopped (optional)
small bunch of chives, finely
    snipped
zest and juice of 1 lemon
sea salt and black pepper

To serve

8 slices of wholemeal bread
sliced cucumber
cress or other micro leaves

Chickpea

400g can of chickpeas, drained
parsley leaves, chopped
zest and juice of 1 lime
2 tsp Dijon mustard
1 tbsp thick yoghurt
½ small red onion, very finely
    chopped
1 celery stick, very finely chopped
1 tbsp finely chopped gherkins
1 tbsp finely chopped black olives
100g sweetcorn, cooked
sea salt and black pepper

To serve

8 slices of wholemeal bread
sliced tomatoes
shredded lettuce or rocket leaves

When you tire of cheese and pickle, here are two new sandwich fillings to spruce up your lunch box – one with fish and one veggie. Both recipes make enough for four regular sandwiches or if you're eating at home, you could make open sandwiches to cut the calories.

SALMON & COTTAGE CHEESE

Put the salmon or tuna, cottage cheese, capers and mustard in a bowl and mix thoroughly. Add the tarragon, if using, most of the chives, the lemon zest and half the juice. Season with pepper (no salt at this stage) and mix thoroughly. Taste and adjust accordingly – you may want to add salt and more lemon juice.

Make your sandwiches with the filling, cucumber slices, a sprinkling of the chives and some cress or other micro leaves.

CHICKPEA

Put the chickpeas, parsley, lime zest and juice, mustard and yoghurt in a food processor and pulse until you have a creamy, green-flecked mixture. Stir in all the remaining ingredients and season with salt and plenty of black pepper.

Make your sandwiches with the filling, sliced tomatoes and lettuce or rocket leaves.

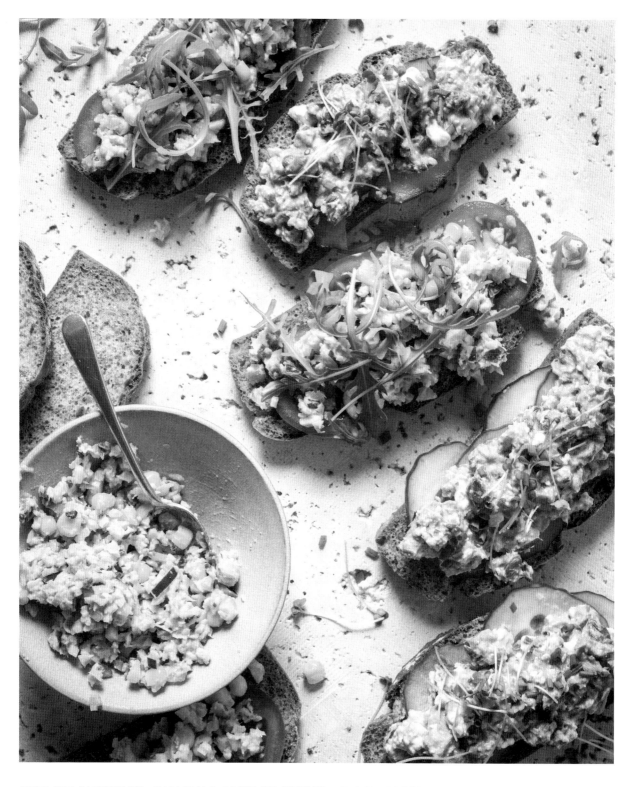

INFO PER SANDWICH: **SALMON & COTTAGE CHEESE:** CALORIES 222 PROTEIN (G) 10 CARBS (G) 29 SUGAR (G) 3 FAT (G) 6 SATURATED FAT (G) 2 FIBRE (G) 5 SALT (G) 1.6
CHICKPEA: CALORIES 287 PROTEIN (G) 13 CARBS (G) 42 SUGAR (G) 4 FAT (G) 5.5 SATURATED FAT (G) 1 FIBRE (G) 9 SALT (G) 1.1

DIPS

Potato & cauliflower skordalia

100g floury potatoes, unpeeled

½ head garlic, cloves unpeeled

200g cauliflower florets

¼–½ tsp turmeric

¼ tsp sugar

100g thick yoghurt or kefir

1 tbsp olive oil

1 tsp red wine vinegar

sea salt and black pepper

Smoked mackerel & beetroot

200g smoked mackerel fillet,
  skinned

1–2 tbsp hot horseradish sauce
  (to taste)

1 small red onion, finely chopped

100g cooked beetroot, coarsely
  grated

1 tbsp apple cider vinegar

fronds from a few sprigs of dill,
  finely chopped

2 tbsp crème fraiche

sea salt and black pepper

It's good to have a tasty dip in the fridge for when hunger strikes or you need something for your lunch box. Skordalia is a Greek dip that's traditionally made with potato, garlic and loads of oil. We've made it lighter by mixing the potato with some cauliflower and cutting back on the oil. The smoked mackerel recipe also works well as a sandwich filling with some cucumber or dill pickles, but if using it this way, don't add the crème fraiche.

POTATO & CAULIFLOWER SKORDALIA

 Prep: **10 minutes**   Cooking time: **about 25 minutes**

Scrub the potatoes well and cut them into chunks. Put them and all but one clove of the garlic cloves in a steamer and cook for 15 minutes. Add the cauliflower and cook for a further 8–10 minutes until very tender. Peel the potatoes and garlic and mash everything together with plenty of salt, half the turmeric and the sugar.

Grate or crush the remaining garlic clove and add it to the mashed vegetables along with the yoghurt or kefir, the olive oil and the red wine vinegar. Beat together until very well combined. Taste and add more seasoning and turmeric if you feel the dip needs it. Serve at room temperature or chilled with raw vegetables or crackers.

SMOKED MACKEREL & BEETROOT

 Prep: **10 minutes**

Put the smoked mackerel into a food processor with a tablespoon of the horseradish and blitz until broken up.

Add the red onion, cooked beetroot and cider vinegar and season with plenty of salt and pepper. Pulse until the ingredients are well combined. Taste and add more horseradish and seasoning if you like. Transfer the mixture to a bowl and stir in the dill. If adding crème fraiche, stir it into the dip just before serving.

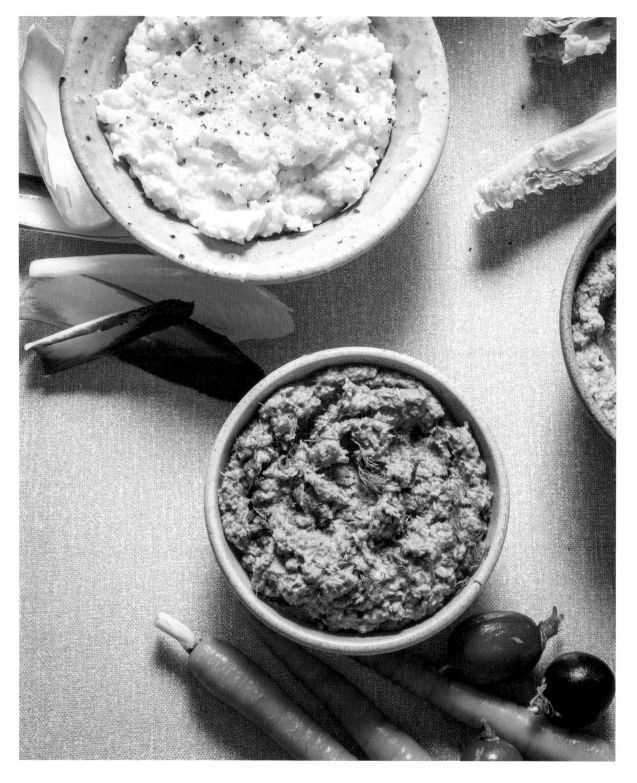

INFO PER SERVING: **POTATO & CAULIFLOWER SKORDALIA** – CALORIES 84 PROTEIN (G) 3 CARBS (G) 9 SUGAR (G) 4 FAT (G) 4 SATURATED FAT (G) 1 FIBRE (G) 1.5 SALT (G) 0.06
SMOKED MACKEREL & BEETROOT (WITH CREME FRAICHE) – CALORIES 211 PROTEIN (G) 11.5 CARBS (G) 6.5 SUGAR (G) 6 FAT (G) 15 SATURATED FAT (G) 4.5 FIBRE (G) 1 SALT (G) 1

MORE DIPS

Baba ganoush

2 large aubergines

1 tsp olive oil

1 tsp oregano

4 fat garlic cloves, unpeeled

1 tbsp tahini

zest and juice of ½ lemon

1 tsp smoked chilli flakes or
    powder, plus extra to garnish

leaves from a few sprigs of mint
    or parsley, roughly chopped

1 tbsp olive oil

sea salt and black pepper

Garnish

1 tsp olive oil

½ preserved lemon, finely
    chopped

Pea & broad bean

175g broad beans (weight before
    skinning)

150g peas or petits pois

3 spring onions, roughly chopped

fronds from a small bunch of dill

½ tsp ground cumin

¼ tsp cinnamon

1 tsp dried mint

zest and juice of 1 lime

50ml quark

To serve

1 tsp olive oil

a squeeze of lime juice

a few dill fronds

*Here are two more of our favourite dips – just the thing
with the Marmite breadsticks on page 82 or some sticks
of raw vegetables.*

BABA GANOUSH

 Prep: **10 minutes**   Cooking time: **about 45 minutes**

Slice the aubergines in half lengthways and cut a cross-hatch pattern
deep into the flesh of each half. No need to peel them – the skins add
flavour and fibre. Preheat the oven to 200°C/Fan 180°C/Gas 6.

Mix the olive oil with a teaspoon of water and brush over the cut sides
of the aubergines. Place the aubergines on a baking tray, cut-side up,
and sprinkle them with the oregano and some salt. Roast in the oven
for 25 minutes. Add the garlic cloves and continue to roast for another
15–20 minutes, until the aubergines are tender and well browned.

Roughly chop the aubergines and put them in a food processor.
Squeeze the flesh from the garlic cloves and add this to the food
processor, together with the tahini, lemon zest and juice, chilli flakes
or powder and most of the mint or parsley. Pulse until you have a thick,
brown-flecked purée, then drizzle in the olive oil until emulsified.

To garnish, mix the olive oil with the preserved lemon and drizzle over
the aubergine purée. Sprinkle over the remaining mint or parsley and
a generous pinch of chilli flakes or powder, then serve.

PEA & BROAD BEAN

 Prep: **10 minutes**   Cooking time: **about 5 minutes**

Cover the broad beans in freshly boiled water and leave them to stand
for a minute. Drain, then peel off the greyish skins and discard them.
Put the beans in a saucepan with the peas or petits pois and cover
with boiling water. Simmer for several minutes until tender. Drain.

Put the spring onions in a small food processor and blitz. Add the
peas, beans and remaining ingredients and process until you have a
fairly smooth purée. Dress with a drizzle of olive oil, a squeeze of lime
and a few more snipped fronds of dill before serving.

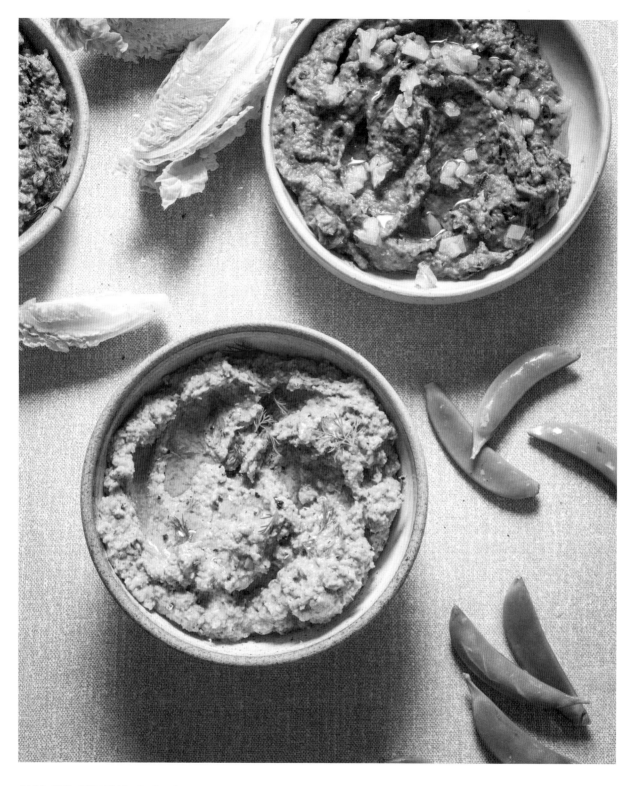

INFO PER SERVING: **BABA GANOUSH** – CALORIES 102   PROTEIN (G) 2.5   CARBS (G) 4.5   SUGAR (G) 3.5
FAT (G) 7   SATURATED FAT (G) 1   FIBRE (G) 5   SALT (G) TRACE
PEA & BROAD BEAN DIP – CALORIES 78   PROTEIN (G) 6   CARBS (G) 7.5   SUGAR (G) 2.5   FAT (G) 2
SATURATED FAT (G) O.5   FIBRE (G)5   SALT (G) TRACE

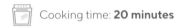
SAUSAGE ROLLS-LIGHT

8 sheets of filo pastry (40 x 30cm)

2 tbsp Dijon mustard or brown
    sauce or onion marmalade

500g sausage meat, or high
    meat-content sausages, skinned

1 egg

1 tbsp milk

1 tbsp sesame and/or nigella seeds

We all love a sausage roll, but they can be a bit high in calories, so we are very happy that we've come up with a lighter version than the regular sort by using filo pastry. Easy to make and pimped up with a dash of mustard or sauce, these really are the business. We like to use Lincolnshire or Cumberland sausages which have plenty of flavour, so you don't need to add much else.

Preheat the oven to 200°C/Fan 180°C/Gas 6. Line a baking tray with baking parchment.

Lay out 4 sheets of the filo pastry on top of one another. Spread a tablespoon of whichever condiment you're using in a line 10cm above the bottom edge of the filo pastry. Take half the sausage meat and squish it together into a long roll. Arrange this over the mustard, brown sauce or onion marmalade.

Beat the egg and milk together, then brush the top layer of filo. Bring the bottom side of this layer over the sausage meat, then roll it up. Brush the next layer of filo pastry and roll that up, then repeat until you have used up all 4 sheets. Brush the surface with more beaten egg and sprinkle with seeds. Cut into 8 pieces.

Arrange the sausage rolls on the baking tray, then repeat with the remaining ingredients so you have 16 sausage rolls. Bake in the preheated oven for 20 minutes until piping hot all the way through and golden brown. Eat hot or cold.

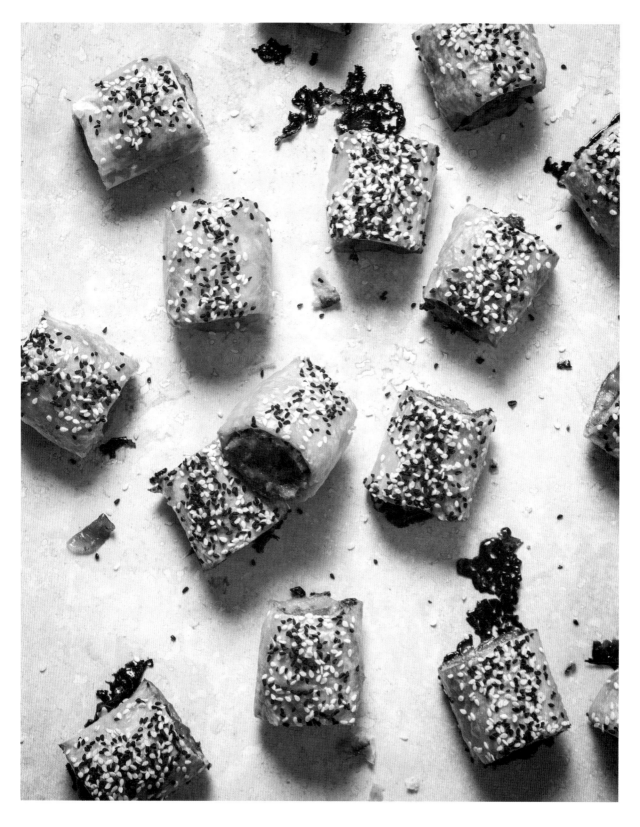

INFO PER ROLL: CALORIES 160   PROTEIN (G) 7   CARBS (G) 14.5   SUGAR (G) 1   FAT (G) 8
SATURATED FAT (G) 2.5   FIBRE (G) 0.8   SALT (G) 0.75

SOUTHERN FRIED CHICKEN

1 tsp garlic powder
1 tsp onion powder
1 tsp dried thyme
1 tsp ground black pepper
200ml buttermilk
1 tsp Worcestershire sauce
8 chicken drumsticks, skinned
75g breadcrumbs
½ tsp sweet smoked paprika
1 tbsp olive oil
sea salt and black pepper

Actually, as you will see, this chicken isn't fried but baked, which means it is way lower in calories and fat but still so good. Chicken drumsticks are cheap and tasty, so are ideal for this recipe, and as they take a while to cook the crumb coating browns and crisps up nicely. You could also use thighs or breasts if you prefer. These are great served with some salad or you can pop them in a lunch box to take to work.

First make the marinade. Put the garlic and onion powders, thyme and black pepper in a large bowl with half a teaspoon of salt, the buttermilk and the Worcestershire sauce. Mix thoroughly.

Make deep slashes in the drumsticks – 3 or 4 in each one – and add them to the buttermilk mixture. Use your hands to massage the buttermilk marinade into the drumsticks so they are well coated, then cover the bowl and put it in the fridge. Leave the chicken to marinate for at least an hour or overnight.

When you are ready to cook the chicken, preheat the oven to 200°C/Fan 180°C/Gas 6 and line a baking tray with baking parchment. Mix the breadcrumbs with the paprika and season with salt and pepper. Dip each drumstick in the breadcrumbs and arrange them on the baking tray. Mix the oil with a tablespoon of water and brush this mixture over the drumsticks.

Bake in the oven for about 40 minutes, turning once or twice during the cooking time.

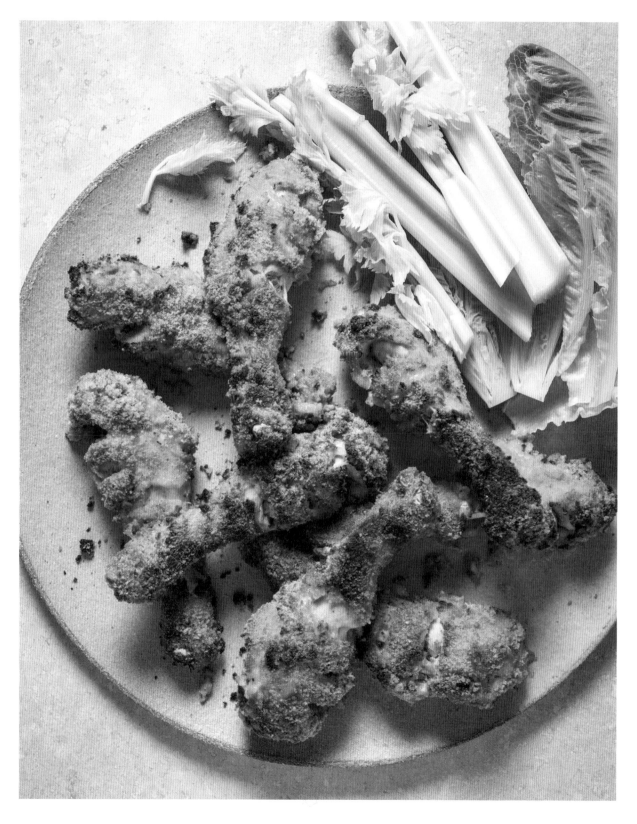

INFO PER SERVING (2 DRUMSTICKS): CALORIES 225 PROTEIN (G) 25 CARBS (G) 17 SUGAR (G) 4 FAT (G) 6 SATURATED FAT (G) 1 FIBRE (G) 0 SALT (G) 0.6

HEART
HE

Y BUT
ALTHY

CHICKEN & CHORIZO TRAY BAKE – 118

VIETNAMESE TURKEY PATTIES – 120

CHICKEN STIR-FRY WITH SATAY SAUCE – 122

BRAISED LAMB WITH GREENS & MASH – 124

LAMB & RICE SALAD – 126

PORK & KIMCHI FRIED RICE – 128

BRAISED AUBERGINES WITH PORK – 130

PORK & LENTIL RISSOLES – 132

STEAK & CANNELLINI BEAN SALAD – 134

SLOW-COOKED FEATHERBLADE – 136

BOILED BEEF WITH CARROTS &
    BEETROOT – 138

MEATBALLS WITH CHIP SHOP
    CURRY SAUCE – 140

AUBERGINE PARMIGIANA

1 tbsp olive oil

3 aubergines, sliced into ½–1cm
   rounds

a few fresh rosemary and oregano
   sprigs

sea salt and black pepper

Sauce

1 tsp olive oil

1 onion, finely chopped

3 garlic cloves, finely chopped

1 tsp dried oregano

generous pinch of cinnamon

400g can of tomatoes

100ml red wine

To assemble

small bunch of basil leaves

2 balls of mozzarella, well drained
   and torn

*This Italian classic is a great favourite of ours, but it's
usually loaded with calories because aubergines soak
up such a huge amount of oil. In this lighter version, we
bake the aubergine slices instead of frying and the result
is just as delicious but much lighter. It's a beautifully
satisfying, comforting dish, so dive in and enjoy.*

Preheat the oven to 200°C/Fan 180°C/Gas 6. Mix the olive oil with
a tablespoon of water. Place the aubergine slices on 2 or 3 baking
trays lined with baking parchment. Brush the slices sparingly with the
olive oil and water mix, then season with salt and pepper. Roughly
break up the sprigs of herbs and sprinkle them over the aubergines.
Bake in the oven for 25–30 minutes until the slices are squidgy in
the middle and nicely browned. Discard the herbs.

While the aubergines are baking, make the sauce. Heat the olive oil
in a saucepan and add the onion. Add a splash of water and sauté the
onion gently until translucent. Add the garlic and continue to sauté for
another 2 or 3 minutes. Sprinkle in the oregano and cinnamon, then
pour the tomatoes and red wine into the pan. Rinse out the can with
100ml of water and add this to the sauce. Season with salt and pepper
and bring the sauce to the boil. Cover and simmer for 10 minutes, then
remove the lid and continue to simmer until the sauce is well reduced.

To assemble, spread a spoonful of the sauce over the base of an
ovenproof dish. Add a layer of aubergines and a couple of torn basil
leaves. Continue until you have used up all the aubergines and sauce,
pressing down well in between each layer.

Add more basil and dot with the torn-up mozzarella. Bake in the oven
for 25–30 minutes until well browned and bubbling.

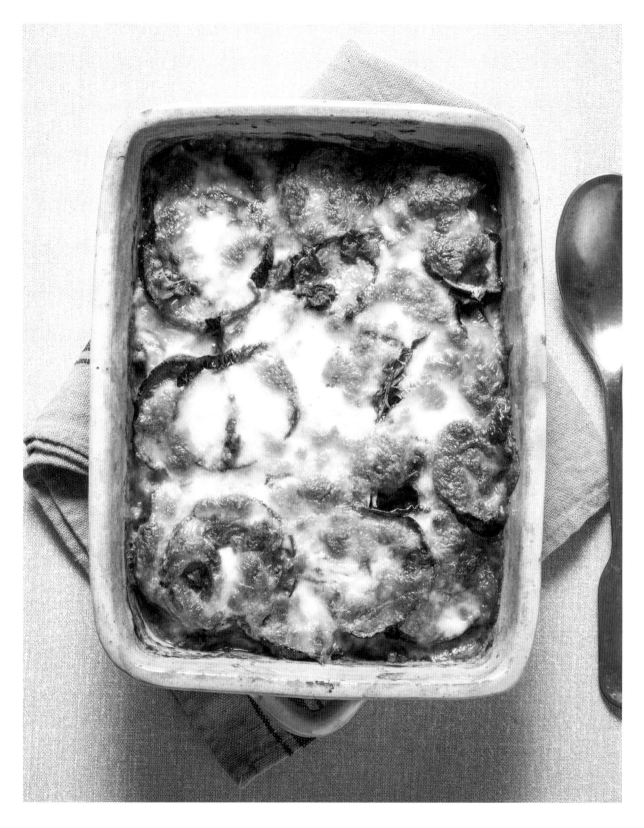

INFO PER SERVING: CALORIES 325   PROTEIN (G) 17.5   CARBS (G) 11   SUGAR (G) 10   FAT (G) 20
SATURATED FAT (G) 11   FIBRE (G) 7.5   SALT (G) 0.8

ROAST CAULIFLOWER & CHICKPEA TRAY BAKE

3 medium onions, cut into
      slim wedges
2 red peppers, cut into strips
1 large cauliflower, cut into
      fairly small florets
1 tbsp olive oil
2 x 400g cans of chickpeas,
      drained
1 tbsp harissa (any sort, the
      smoked chilli one is good)
sea salt and black pepper

Sauce
large bunch of coriander,
      roughly chopped
1 garlic clove, finely chopped
1 or 2 green chillies, finely
      chopped
zest and juice of 1 lemon
1 tbsp tahini
50g plain yoghurt

Garnish
1 tsp za'atar
a few mint leaves

Lots of zesty flavours bring this dish together. Cauliflower is a great choice for a low-calorie but filling meal and this tray bake is a real treat. The chickpeas add some bulk and fibre and the tahini sauce, pepped up with za'atar, is a delight. Za'atar, by the way is a Middle Eastern spice mix that's become very popular and is available in most supermarkets now. Serve the dish with some steamed greens on the side, if you like.

Preheat the oven to 200°C/Fan 180°C/Gas 6.

To make the sauce, put all the ingredients except the yoghurt into a food processor or blender and season with salt and pepper. Blitz until you have a green-flecked sauce, then stir in the yoghurt. The sauce will thicken as it is left to stand.

Put the onions, red peppers and cauliflower florets in a large roasting tin. Mix the olive oil with a tablespoon of water and drizzle over the vegetables. Stir to coat the veg in the oil and season with salt and black pepper.

Roast the vegetables in the oven for 25 minutes, turning them over once during that time.

Put the chickpeas in a bowl. Mix the harissa with a little water, then add this and a little salt to the chickpeas and toss well. Add the chickpeas to the roasting tin and give everything a good shake. Roast for a further 5–10 minutes until the vegetables are completely tender and lightly charred.

To serve, sprinkle with za'atar and a few mint leaves and drizzle with the sauce.

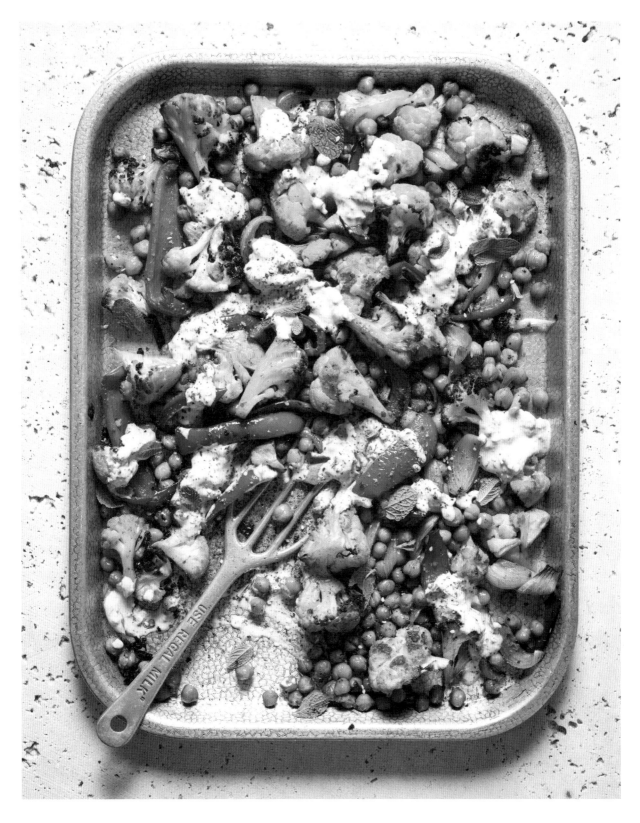

INFO PER SERVING: CALORIES 364 PROTEIN (G) 17.5 CARBS (G) 41 SUGAR (G) 17 FAT (G) 11
SATURATED FAT (G) 2 FIBRE (G) 16 SALT (G) TRACE

BLACK-EYED BEANS WITH HALLOUMI

1 tbsp olive oil
1 red onion, finely diced
1 red pepper, finely diced
1 courgette, diced
3 garlic cloves, finely chopped
1 tsp dried oregano
zest and juice of 1 lemon
2 x 400g cans of black-eyed
    beans, drained
1 medium or large tomato, diced
1 tsp red wine vinegar
1 small bunch of dill, finely
    chopped
1 small bunch of parsley,
    finely chopped
sea salt and black pepper

To serve
250g block of halloumi, cut
    into 8 slices
juice of 1 lemon
a few mint leaves, finely chopped
pinch of chilli flakes (optional)

Also known as black-eyed peas, these tasty little beans have a great flavour and texture which works well in this dish. Topped with crispy, salty halloumi, this hits the spot for an easy, filling veggie supper. Use canned beans or soak and cook your own if you prefer.

Heat the olive oil in a wide-based pan. Add the onion, pepper and courgette and cook gently until the onion is translucent but still has a little bite to it. Add the garlic and cook for another couple of minutes, then add the oregano and lemon zest.

Roughly mash about one third of the beans to break them up a bit, then add them and the whole ones to the pan of vegetables. Season with salt and pepper. Add the lemon juice, tomato and wine vinegar and about 50ml of water, then simmer until the beans are just heated through. The vegetables should still have some crunch to them.

Stir in the herbs, then taste and add any more seasoning or lemon juice to get the flavour you like.

Heat a griddle pan until it's too hot to hold your hand over. Add the halloumi slices and grill them for a couple of minutes until the cheese comes away cleanly and is marked with deep char lines on the underside. Flip over and repeat, then transfer the slices to a plate and dress with lemon juice, mint and chilli flakes. Serve with the beans.

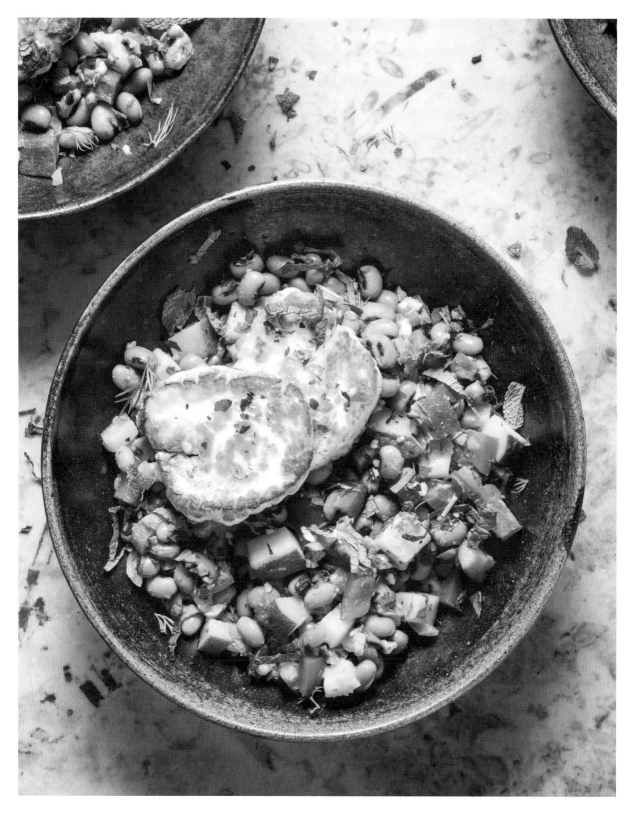

INFO PER SERVING: CALORIES 400   PROTEIN (G) 25.5   CARBS (G) 29   SUGAR (G) 8   FAT (G) 18.5
SATURATED FAT (G) 11   FIBRE (G) 8   SALT (G) 2

GREEK BAKED VEGETABLES

600g new potatoes, thickly sliced

3 red onions, sliced into wedges

2 red peppers, cut into strips

1 green pepper, cut into strips

2 courgettes, cut into 2cm slices
   on the diagonal

1 tbsp olive oil

2 tsp red wine vinegar

a few fresh oregano sprigs

50ml white wine

100g fresh tomatoes, roughly
   chopped

3 garlic cloves, roughly chopped

pinch of cinnamon

½ tsp dried mint

50g olives, pitted

200g feta cheese, cut into small
   cubes (optional)

sea salt and black pepper

This is our low-cal version of a wonderful Greek dish known as briam. There are loads of different regional variations, but our recipe has much less olive oil than usual, so keeps the calories down. It makes a great supper dish with a green salad and, if you want to make it more substantial, add some cubes of feta cheese. Or it would make a lovely side dish to some barbecued lamb.

Preheat the oven to 200°C/Fan 180°C/Gas 6. Bring a pan of water to the boil, add the potato slices and cook for 3 or 4 minutes, then drain.

Put the potatoes and other vegetables in a roasting tin or ovenproof dish and season with salt and pepper. Whisk the olive oil and red wine vinegar together and drizzle the mixture over the vegetables. Mix thoroughly, then add the fresh oregano. Roast in the oven for about 20 minutes.

Put the white wine, tomatoes, garlic, cinnamon and mint in a small food processor or blender and whizz to a purée. Take the dish out of the oven and pour this around the vegetables. Add the olives and continue to bake for another 25–30 minutes until the vegetables are tender and browning around the edges.

If you want to include feta, add it to the vegetables for the last 5 minutes of the cooking time.

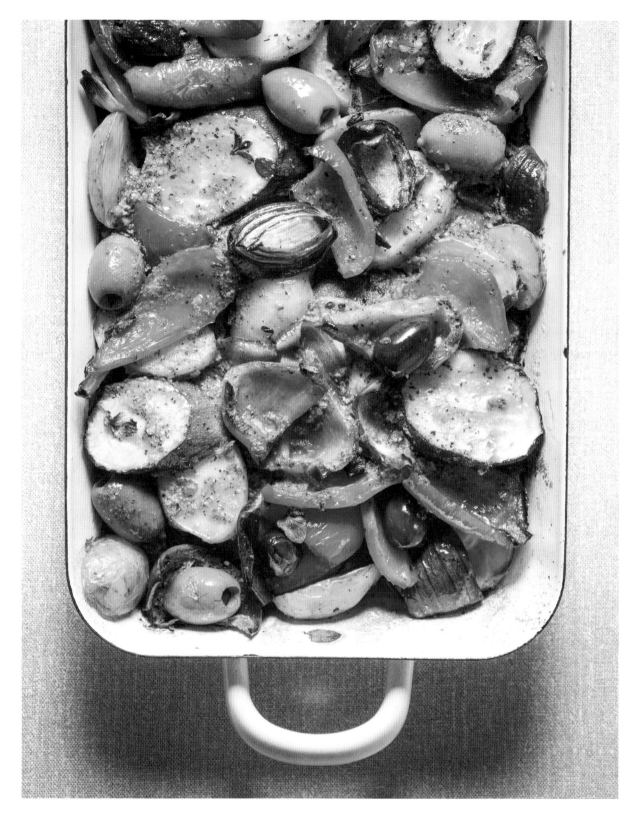

INFO PER SERVING/WITH FETA: CALORIES 276/400   PROTEIN (G) 6/14   CARBS (G) 40/41
SUGAR (G) 14.5/15   FAT (G) 7/17   SATURATED FAT (G) 1/8   FIBRE (G) 9/9   SALT (G) TRACE/1.64

COURGETTE POVERELLA WITH ORECCHIETTE

3 large courgettes, sliced into rounds
1 tbsp olive oil
4 garlic cloves, finely sliced
leaves from a small bunch of mint, finely chopped
3–4 tsp white balsamic vinegar
400g orecchiette
sea salt and black pepper

Dishes cooked 'alla poverella' are Italian classics and the term refers to recipes that are simple and inexpensive but always so good to eat. Orecchiette are a traditional pasta shape from southern Italy and look like little ears. They work beautifully with the silky-soft braised courgettes in this recipe. Ideally, salt the courgettes first as described below to get rid of excess liquid and reduce bitterness. Usually, the courgettes for this dish are fried in lots of oil but braising them over a low heat with the minimum of oil gives excellent results. If you don't have white balsamic vinegar, use white wine vinegar with a good pinch of sugar mixed into it.

First, if you have time, salt the courgettes. Put them in a large colander and sprinkle them with a teaspoon of salt. Leave for at least half an hour, preferably an hour, then drain on a tea towel or kitchen paper.

Heat the olive oil in a large, lidded sauté pan. Add the garlic and cook over a gentle heat for a couple of minutes, then add the courgettes. Stir for a further couple of minutes or until the courgettes are giving off steam, then cover and leave over a low heat for a few minutes, stirring regularly, until the courgettes are tender. Stir in the mint, reserving a few sprigs for the garnish, and sprinkle in the balsamic vinegar a teaspoon at a time, tasting as you go – it doesn't add a distinct flavour but just rounds off the dish nicely.

While the courgettes are braising, cook the orecchiette in plenty of boiling, salted water. When al dente, remove a ladleful of the cooking liquid, then drain the pasta in a colander. Add the pasta to the pan with the courgettes and stir until well combined. If it looks at all dry, add a little of the reserved cooking water. Serve with plenty of black pepper and the reserved mint leaves.

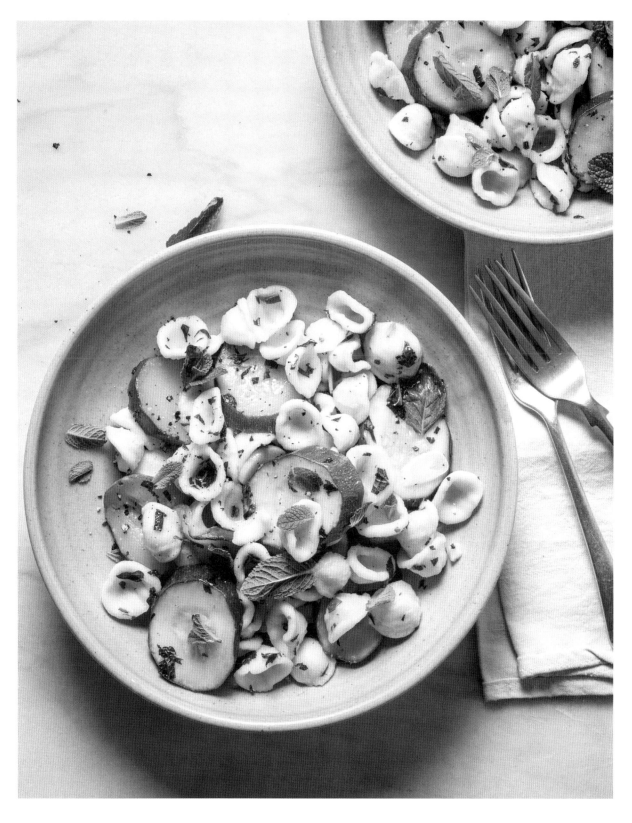

INFO PER SERVING: CALORIES 417   PROTEIN (G) 15   CARBS (G) 75   SUGAR (G) 4   FAT (G) 5
SATURATED FAT (G) 1   FIBRE (G) 7   SALT (G) TRACE

SPICED FISH & SALSA

4 fish fillets, such as snapper,
    sea bass or bream, skinned
1 tsp melted butter or olive oil
zest of 1 lime
sea salt

Rub
1 tsp dried thyme
½ tsp garlic powder
½ tsp onion powder
½ tsp ground allspice
½ tsp cayenne
½ tsp ground black pepper

Cucumber & mango salsa
½ cucumber, deseeded and
    finely diced
1 fairly firm mango, peeled,
    stoned and finely diced
½ red pepper, finely diced
½ scotch bonnet, deseeded
    and very finely diced
zest and juice of 1 lime
a few basil or parsley leaves,
    shredded

Fish is high in protein and nutrients but low in calories. This dish is inspired by a dish we cooked in a bikers' bar in the Ozarks on our 'Route 66' adventure. Little did we realise that our new healthy version would taste just as good. A nice firm-fleshed fish, such as snapper, is best for this – you need something that doesn't flake too easily. The salsa works beautifully with the fish, as does a dish of rice and peas, or you could just opt for some green veg instead of the rice for a lower-calorie meal.

Preheat the oven to 200°C/Fan 180°C/Gas 6 and line a baking tray with baking parchment.

For the salsa, cut the cucumber in half lengthways and remove the seeds with a spoon, then dice the flesh. Mix the cucumber with all the other salsa ingredients and a generous pinch of salt and leave to stand until the fish is ready.

Mix all the rub ingredients together. Sprinkle the fish fillets with salt, followed by a light dusting of the rub, making sure you cover both sides of each fillet. Mix the melted butter or oil with the lime zest and a teaspoon of water. Dab this over the fish fillets.

Place the fish on a baking tray and roast it in the oven for 12–15 minutes until cooked through. Lovely served with the salsa and some rice and peas (see page 173).

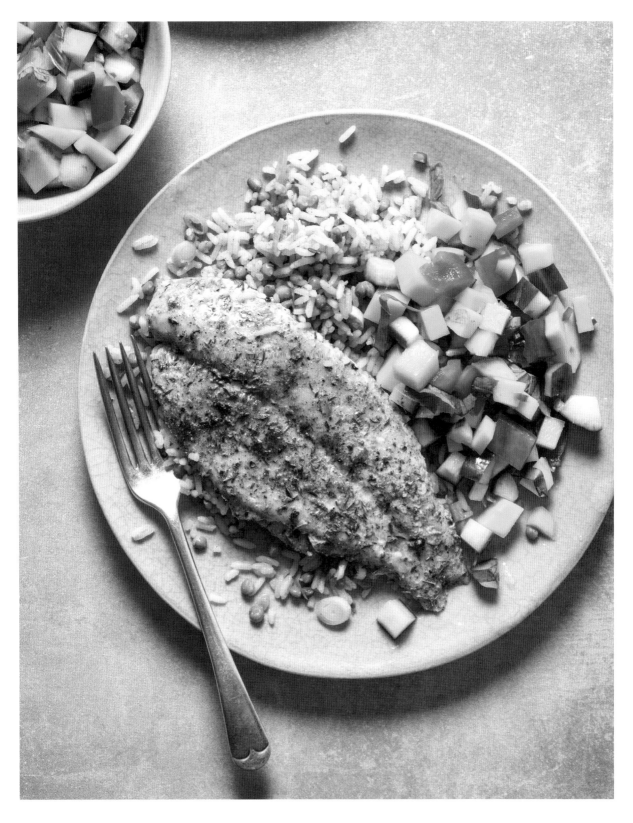

INFO PER SERVING (SPICED FISH AND SALSA):   CALORIES 313   PROTEIN (G) 31   CARBS (G) 10
SUGAR (G) 9   FAT (G) 16   SATURATED FAT (G) 4   FIBRE (G) 3   SALT (G) TRACE

FISH BITE TACOS

1 tsp ground cumin
½ tsp ground cinnamon
½ tsp ground allspice
¼ – ½ tsp chilli powder
   (chipotle is good)
500g firm, white fish fillet,
   cut into 2–3cm chunks
sea salt and black pepper

Salsa
zest and juice of 1 lime
½ tsp salt
½ red onion, finely diced
4 tomatoes, finely diced
1–2 jalapeños, finely diced
2 tbsp finely chopped coriander
   stems and leaves

To serve
8 corn tortillas
coriander sprigs
pickled jalapeños (optional)

We've kept these nice and simple and made the little morsels of fish super-flavoursome so you don't need all the usual taco extras like cheese and soured cream. But if you do want to add any extra bits and bobs, that's up to you and your waistline. Zesty and tasty – a real treat.

Preheat the oven to 200°C/Fan 180°C/Gas 6. Line a baking tray with baking parchment.

Make the salsa. Put the lime zest and juice in a bowl with the salt. Add the red onion and leave it to marinate for about half an hour – this will help soften the flavour and intensify the colour. Add the remaining ingredients, taste for seasoning and adjust if necessary. Leave to stand at room temperature.

For the fish, mix all the spices together with plenty of salt and pepper. Toss the fish in the spices, then arrange the pieces on the baking tray, spacing them out well. Bake in the oven for 10 minutes, then remove.

Heat the corn tortillas and serve the fish with the tortillas, salsa and pickled jalapeños, if using.

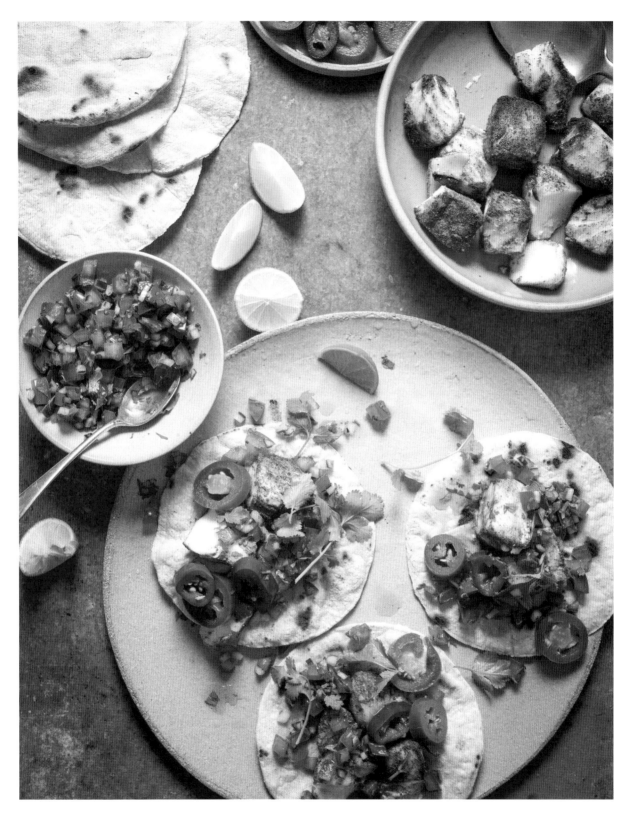

INFO PER SERVING: CALORIES 363   PROTEIN (G) 28   CARBS (G) 49   SUGAR (G) 6   FAT (G) 5
SATURATED FAT (G) 1   FIBRE (G) 3   SALT (G) 1.6

PRAWN & SALMON BURGERS

400g salmon fillet
180g raw peeled prawns
3 spring onions, finely chopped
2 tsp sushi ginger, very finely
    chopped
1 tbsp tamari or soy sauce
1 tsp sesame seeds (preferably
    black)
1 tsp sesame oil
sea salt and black pepper

Pickled cucumber
1 large cucumber
1 tsp sugar
1 tbsp Japanese rice vinegar
1 tsp wasabi paste

To serve
4 burger buns or 4 large lettuce
    leaves
watercress sprigs

These taste very rich and luxurious, but happily, oily fish like salmon is good for us and these burgers make a delicious and filling meal. The Japanese-style pickled cucumber is the perfect accompaniment, cutting through the richness beautifully. Serve the burgers on lettuce leaves if you're watching the calories or on burger buns, or try our cloud bread on page 32 for a change.

First prepare the pickled cucumber. Cut the cucumber in half lengthways and remove the seeds with a spoon – no need to peel. Using a vegetable peeler, slice the cucumber into ribbons. Put the cucumber ribbons in a colander and sprinkle with a teaspoon of salt, then place over a bowl and leave to stand for half an hour. The cucumber will give out plenty of liquid which will drain into the bowl.

Squeeze the cucumber ribbons gently, then transfer them to a tea towel or some kitchen paper to blot off any excess liquid. Whisk the sugar, vinegar and wasabi paste together in a large bowl and add the cucumber. Toss gently to combine. Taste for seasoning and add a little salt if you think it needs it.

Now make the burgers. Preheat the oven to 180°C/Fan 160°C/Gas 4. Put two-thirds of the salmon and peeled prawns in a food processor, then blitz for a few seconds until puréed. Finely chop the remaining salmon and prawns – this will give the burger some texture. Transfer both the puréed and the chopped salmon and prawns to a bowl and add the spring onions, sushi ginger, tamari or soy sauce and the sesame seeds. Mix well and season with a little salt and pepper. Shape into 4 burgers.

Place the burgers on a baking tray. Mix the sesame oil with 2 teaspoons of water and brush the burgers. Bake for 15 minutes. Lightly toast the burger buns, if using, and serve the burgers with plenty of the cucumber and a few sprigs of watercress.

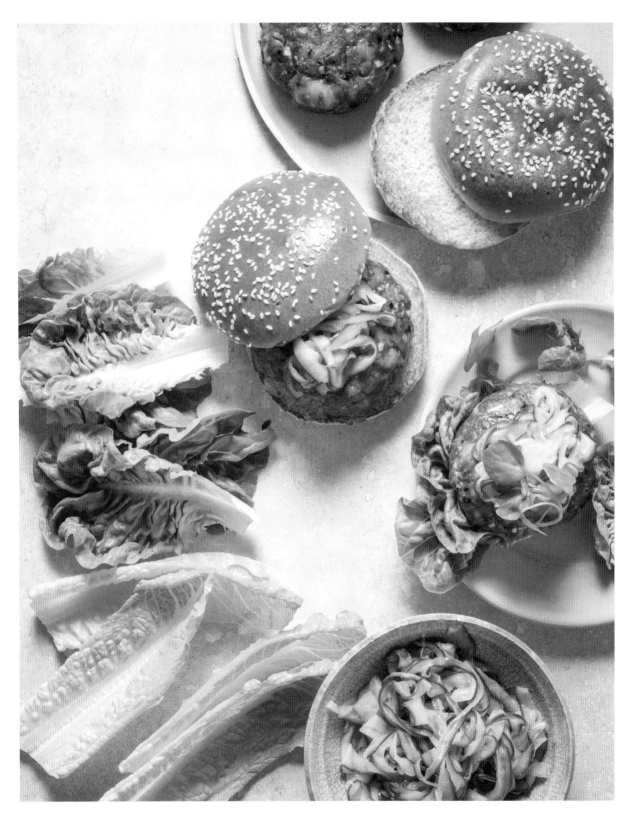

INFO PER SERVING/WITH BUN: CALORIES 295/460   PROTEIN (G) 30/35   CARBS (G) 4/32
SUGAR (G) 3.5/4.5   FAT (G) 17.5/20.5   SATURATED FAT (G) 3/4   FIBRE (G) 1.5/2.5 SALT (G) 0.95/1.9

CHICKEN & MUSHROOM ALFREDO

Sauce

1 tbsp olive oil
1 large onion, finely chopped
2 chicken thigh fillets, skinned and thinly sliced
400g mushrooms (white or chestnut), sliced
3 garlic cloves, finely chopped
leaves from a sprig of oregano
50ml white wine or vermouth
50g quark or similar
50ml crème fraiche
sea salt and black pepper

Pasta

200g tagliatelle or linguine
large head of broccoli, cut into florets
25g Parmesan, grated (optional)

Pasta alfredo is a classic dish, but it's usually mega rich in cream, cheese and butter and so is high in calories. We've come up with a new, low-cal version that's still lovely and creamy and full of flavour from the chicken, mushrooms and broccoli. And all this means that you can cut right back on the pasta. It's a win-win.

Heat the olive oil in a large sauté pan. Add the onion and sauté gently until it's soft and translucent, stirring regularly. Turn up the heat a little and add the chicken and mushrooms. Continue to sauté until the chicken is just cooked through and the mixture is quite dry. Stir in the garlic and oregano and season with salt and pepper.

Pour in the white wine or vermouth and bring to the boil. When the alcohol has evaporated away, stir in the quark and crème fraiche to make a creamy sauce.

Meanwhile, bring a large pan of water to the boil and add salt. Add the pasta and cook for about 8 minutes, then add the broccoli. Cook for another 3–4 minutes or until the pasta and broccoli are just al dente.

Drain the pasta and broccoli, reserving a ladleful of the cooking water. Add about 100ml of the cooking water to the sauce to loosen it and stir over a gentle heat for a couple of minutes until it thickens slightly. Add the pasta and broccoli to the pan and toss until it's all well coated with the sauce. Serve with grated Parmesan, if you like.

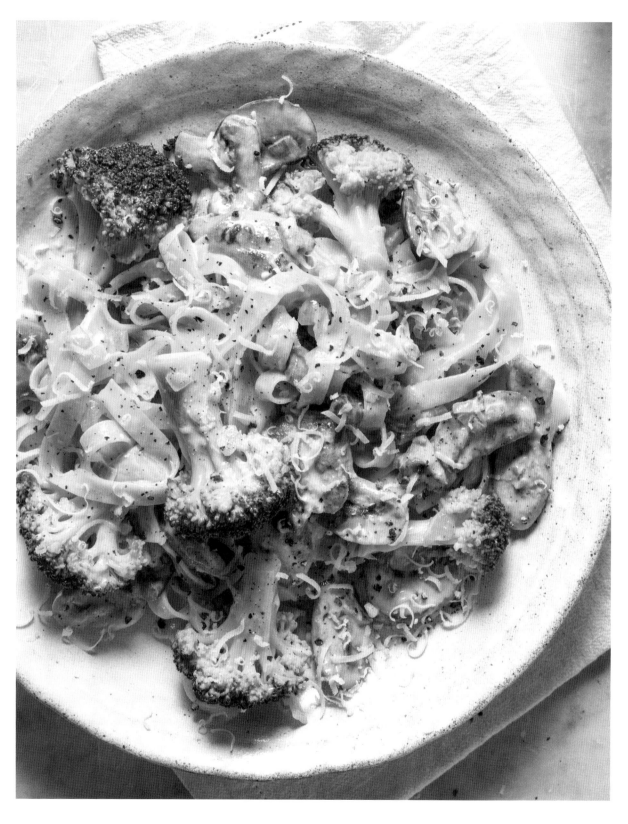

INFO PER SERVING/WITH CHEESE: CALORIES 386/412   PROTEIN (G) 25/27.5   CARBS (G) 45/45
SUGAR (G) 7.5/7.5   FAT (G) 8/10   SATURATED FAT (G) 2.5/3.5   FIBRE (G) 9/9   SALT (G) TRACE/TRACE

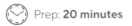

CHICKEN & WHITE BEAN CHILLI

2 tsp olive oil
1 onion, finely chopped
1 green pepper, finely chopped
2 celery sticks, finely chopped
4 garlic cloves, finely chopped
2 or 3 jalapeños or any medium-
  hot chillies, finely chopped
small bunch of coriander, stems
  and leaves separated and
  finely chopped
1 tsp ground cumin
1 tsp ground coriander
¼ tsp each of ground allspice,
  cinnamon and cloves
1 tsp dried oregano
2 bay leaves
3 x 400g cans of cannellini beans
750ml chicken stock
300g cooked chicken breast,
  skinned and diced
100g cream cheese or quark
juice of 1 lime
sea salt and black pepper

To serve (optional)
1 avocado, diced and tossed
  in lime juice
50g hard cheese such as
  Cheddar, grated
pickled jalapeños
warm tortillas

We love a chilli and this recipe is very different from the usual tomato-based version. It's much lighter but still tastes rich and delicious and we add creaminess with just a little quark or cream cheese and a small amount of grated Cheddar on top. The sauce is thickened by mashing some of the beans. You could serve this with rice, but we prefer avocado, chillies and tortillas.

Heat the olive oil in a large pan and add the onion, pepper and celery. Sauté for several minutes until they start to soften, then add the garlic, jalapeños and coriander stems. Sauté for few minutes more, then stir in the spices, oregano and bay leaves.

Take 150g of the cannellini beans and mash them roughly. Add them to the pan along with the whole beans, then cover with the chicken stock. Season with salt and pepper and bring to the boil, then turn down the heat and cover the pan. Simmer for 10 minutes, then add the chicken and the cream cheese or quark.

Stir over a very gentle heat until the chicken is heated through and the cream cheese or quark has dissolved into the sauce. Taste for seasoning and add half the lime juice. Stir and taste – add the remaining lime juice if you think it needs it.

Serve the chilli garnished with fresh coriander leaves and the optional extra if you like.

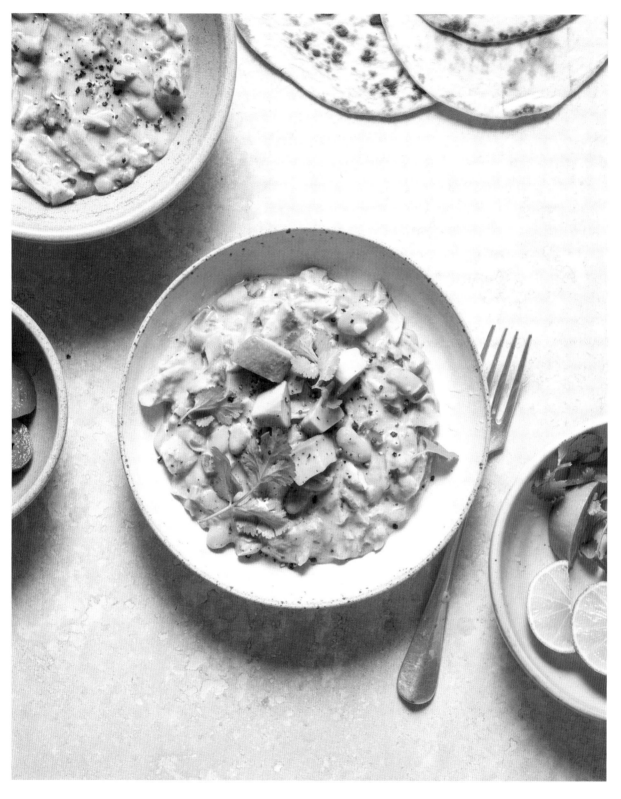

INFO PER SERVING/WITH SERVING SUGGESTIONS: CALORIES 432/767   PROTEIN (G) 40/50
CARBS (G 35.5/72   SUGAR (G) 5/7   FAT (G) 11/26.5   SATURATED FAT (G) 4/11   FIBRE (G) 15/19
SALT (G) TRACE/1.8

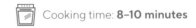
CHICKEN SHAWARMA

2 large skinless, boneless
   chicken breasts
zest and juice of 1 lemon
2 garlic cloves, crushed
1 tsp ground cumin
½ tsp ground coriander
¼ tsp cinnamon
¼ tsp ground allspice
¼ tsp cayenne
½ tsp dried oregano
1 tsp olive oil
sea salt and black pepper

Yoghurt dip
200g plain yoghurt or thick kefir
1 tsp dried mint
pinch of sugar
½ tsp sumac

To serve
4 large lettuce leaves or flatbreads
½ cucumber, sliced
a few pickled chillies (optional)

Traditionally, shawarma is a slow-cooked dish, but slicing chicken breasts in half like this and batting them out to make two much thinner pieces makes them go further and cook super quickly. The spicy yoghurt marinade and the short cooking time keeps the flesh lovely and tender and juicy. What's not to love?

First cut the chicken breasts in half as if you were butterflying them. To do this, put the chicken breast on the work surface and slice through it from one long side to the other. Cut all the way through so you have 2 pieces with the same surface area but half the thickness. Put each piece between 2 pieces of cling film and pound them with a mallet until they are just ½ cm thick. Repeat with the other breast.

Put the lemon zest and juice, garlic, spices, oregano and olive oil into a bowl with plenty of salt and pepper. Mix thoroughly, then add the chicken and rub the mixture into it. Leave to marinate for a few hours if possible, or overnight.

To cook the chicken, heat a dry frying pan or a griddle pan. When it's hot, add the chicken breasts and cook on one side until they are well browned and lift off easily with no sticking. Cook the other side for another 2–3 minutes. Check the chicken is cooked through, then remove from the pan.

For the dressing, mix the yoghurt or kefir, mint and sugar together with a pinch of salt, then sprinkle with the sumac. Serve the chicken on lettuce leaves or flatbreads with the cucumber, dressing and pickled chillies, if using.

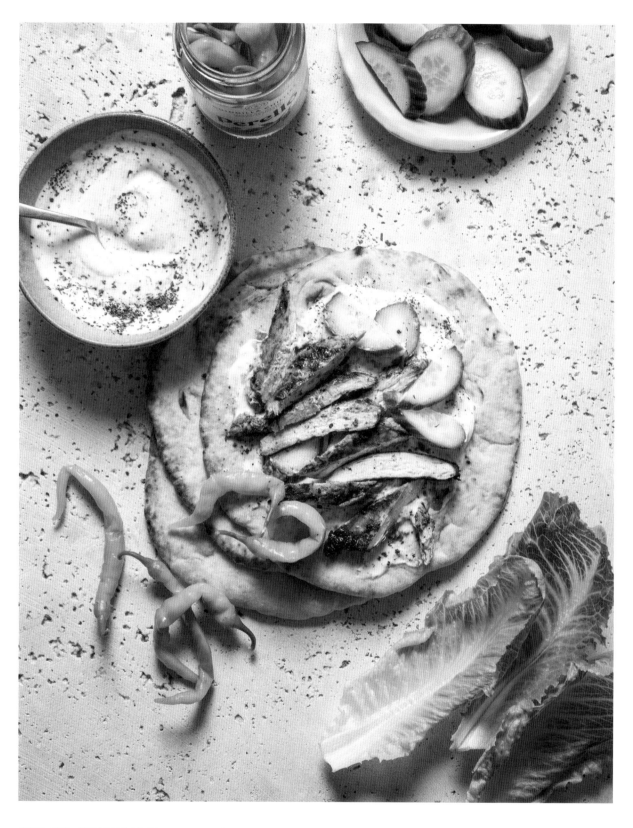

INFO PER SERVING WITH LETTUCE/WITH FLATBREAD: CALORIES 153/363 PROTEIN (G) 27/33 CARBS (G) 4/38 SUGAR (G) 4/6 FAT (G) 3/8 SATURATED FAT (G) 1.5/2 FIBRE (G) 0/2 SALT (G) TRACE/0.8

CHICKEN & CHORIZO TRAY BAKE

100g cooking chorizo, sliced

4 chicken thigh fillets, skinned and halved

3 leeks, cut into rounds

1 large or 2 medium courgettes, sliced into rounds

300g baby new or salad potatoes, halved

50ml chicken stock or water

50ml white wine

4 little gem lettuces, trimmed and halved

200g broad beans

leaves from a few mint sprigs, finely chopped

sea salt and black pepper

Everyone loves a tray bake and this one is no exception. It's so simple to put together, then you just stick it in the oven and you have a cracking dinner. Chicken and chorizo are always a great combo and here they are bulked out with loads of lovely veg. You don't need extra oil, as the chorizo provides plenty, plus lots of flavour. We're sure this recipe will become a family favourite.

Preheat the oven to 200°C/Fan 180°C/Gas 6. Put the chorizo, chicken, leeks, courgettes and potatoes into a large roasting tin and season with salt and pepper. Pour over the chicken stock or water and the white wine, then cover the tin with foil and bake in the oven for 30 minutes.

Remove from the oven and take off the foil. Stir well to coat everything in the oil released from the chorizo. Rub the cut side of the little gems on the base of the roasting tin so they pick up some oil, then tuck them in with the other vegetables, cut-side up. Roast, uncovered, for a further 20 minutes until everything has taken on some colour and is tender to the point of a knife.

Before the end of the cooking time, cook the broad beans in plenty of boiling water, then toss them with the mint and mix into the roasting tin before serving.

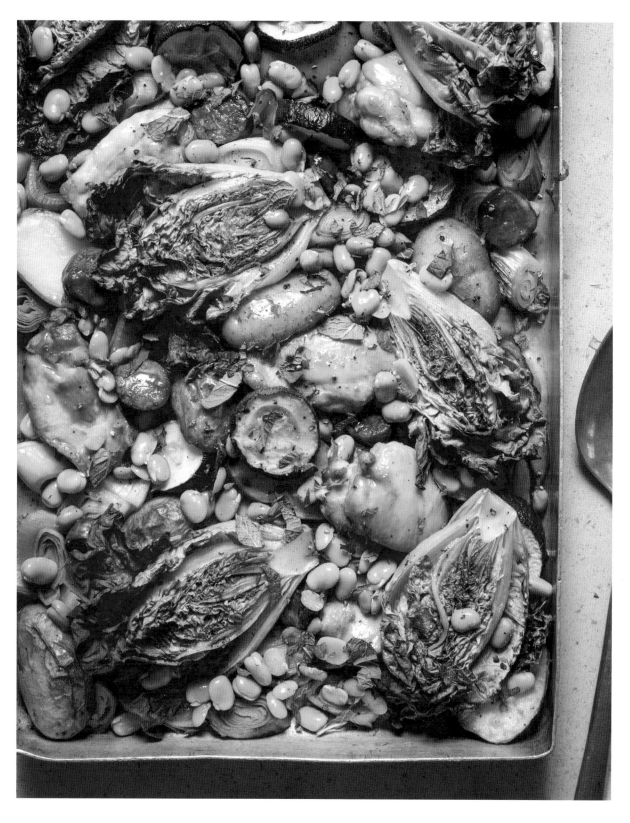

INFO PER SERVING: CALORIES 335   PROTEIN (G) 30   CARBS (G) 20   SUGAR (G) 6   FAT (G) 12
SATURATED FAT (G) 4   FIBRE (G) 11   SALT (G) 1.2

VIETNAMESE TURKEY PATTIES

400g turkey or chicken mince
2 spring onions, very finely chopped
2 garlic cloves, finely chopped
zest of 1 lime
1 lemongrass stalk, white centre only, finely chopped
1 tbsp fish sauce
1 tbsp kecap manis
sea salt and black pepper

Glaze
1 tbsp kecap manis
1 tsp runny honey

Dressing
3 tbsp fish sauce
2 tbsp rice wine vinegar
juice of 1 lime
1 tsp runny honey
1–2 bird's eye chillies, very finely chopped

To serve
150g runner or helda beans, shredded
2 nests of vermicelli rice noodles (optional)
1 large carrot, coarsely grated
1 floppy lettuce, torn into large pieces
½ cucumber, cut into sticks
100g bean sprouts
50g radishes, sliced
small bunch of mint leaves

This is our version of a traditional Vietnamese dish of caramelised patties or meatballs, known as bun cha. It's usually made with pork, but we're using turkey or chicken mince instead, which keeps the dish low in calories but still proper tasty. You could add any kind of cooked greens, such as sprouting or regular broccoli, kale or Chinese greens. Kecap manis is an Indonesian sauce that's a bit like soy sauce but sweeter and more syrupy in texture. You can buy it in big supermarkets.

First make the patties. Preheat the oven to 200°C/Fan 180°C/Gas 6 and line a baking tray with baking parchment.

If the mince is very coarse, blitz it briefly in a food processor. Add all the remaining patty ingredients and season with salt and pepper. Mix thoroughly – the mixture will seem quite soft to start with but if you knead it for a couple of minutes, it will hold together better. Form into 12 patties – if you do this with wet hands the patties will be less sticky and you will get a smoother finish.

Place the patties on the baking tray. Mix the kecap manis with the honey and brush over the top of the patties. Bake them in the oven for 12–15 minutes, until they are cooked through and are lightly caramelised on top.

Meanwhile, blanch the beans in a pan of boiling water for a couple of minutes, then refresh them under cold water. Cook the rice noodles, if using, according to the packet instructions.

Whisk the dressing ingredients together, making sure the honey completely dissolves. Season with salt and pepper.

Divide the beans and other vegetables and the noodles, if using, between 4 bowls. Drizzle over the dressing, then top with the patties and a few mint leaves.

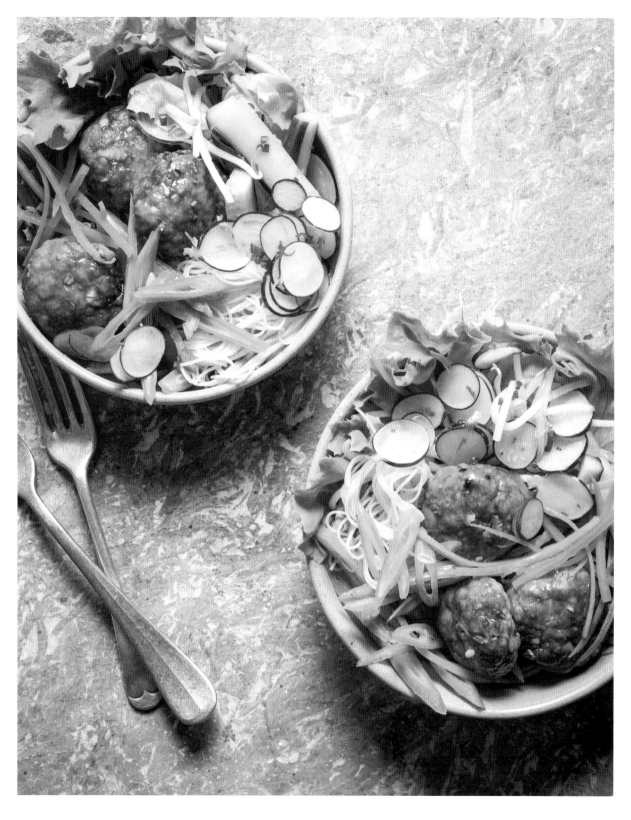

INFO PER SERVING/WITH NOODLES: CALORIES 205/343   PROTEIN (G) 26/30   CARBS (G) 13/41
SUGAR (G) 11/11   FAT (G) 5/5   SATURATED FAT (G) 1.5/1.5   FIBRE (G) 4/4.5   SALT (G) 1.95/1.95

CHICKEN STIR-FRY WITH SATAY SAUCE

2 skinless, boneless chicken
    breasts
1 heaped tsp cornflour
1 tbsp rice wine vinegar
pinch of sugar
sea salt and black pepper

Satay sauce
100ml chicken or vegetable stock
10g root ginger, finely chopped
2 garlic cloves, finely chopped
1 tbsp lime juice
1 tbsp soy sauce
1 tsp runny honey
2 tbsp peanut butter
    (smooth or crunchy)
1–2 tsp hot sauce
    (such as Sriracha)

Stir-fry
2 tsp vegetable oil
1 shallot, finely sliced
100g green cabbage, shredded
200g asparagus spears, trimmed
    and cut into sections
100g mangetout, trimmed and
    sliced at an angle
100g baby corn, halved
    lengthways at an angle

With plenty of veg and protein, this is the perfect quick supper for two people – really good fast food. It could also be served with rice or noodles if you like. The satay sauce is a cracker and the whole dish will delight your taste buds.

First cut the chicken into thin strips. Mix the cornflour with the rice wine vinegar and add salt and a pinch of sugar. Toss the chicken in this mixture and leave it to marinate for at least half an hour.

Next make the sauce. Put all the ingredients in a small saucepan and heat, whisking to make sure the peanut butter combines into a smooth sauce. Taste for seasoning and add more soy sauce or honey to taste.

When you are ready to cook, bring a saucepan of water to the boil. Add the chicken and blanch for just a minute – it will cook pretty much instantly. Drain thoroughly.

Heat a teaspoon of oil in a wok. When it is smoking hot, add the chicken and stir-fry until it is lightly brown. Remove from the wok with a slotted spoon.

Heat the remaining oil, again until smoking. Add the vegetables and stir-fry until they are cooked but still have some bite – this will take just a few minutes. Return the chicken to the wok and pour over the sauce. Cook until everything is piping hot and serve immediately.

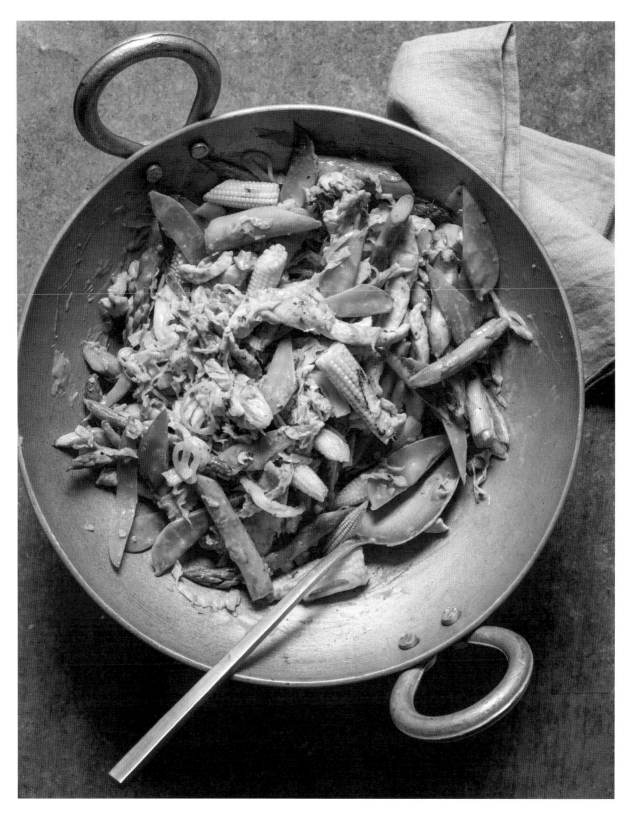

INFO PER SERVING: CALORIES 510   PROTEIN (G) 40   CARBS (G) 23   SUGAR (G) 15   FAT (G) 22
SATURATED FAT (G) 4   FIBRE (G) 8.5   SALT (G) 1.7

BRAISED LAMB WITH GREENS & MASH

4 lamb steaks, trimmed of all fat
    (about 500g)
1 small tin of anchovies
1 large onion, finely sliced
cloves from a bulb of garlic,
    peeled and left whole
a few rosemary sprigs
100ml red wine
large bunch of cavolo nero
    or similar, shredded
squeeze of lemon juice
sea salt and black pepper

Mash
1 large swede, about 750g, diced
4 large carrots, diced
1 tbsp wholegrain mustard
1 tbsp crème fraiche

This makes a really warming, comforting meal. Surprising though it might seem, lamb and anchovies are a classic combo – the anchovies add a good savoury quality to the dish but there's no fishy taste.

First heat a griddle pan until it is very hot. Season the lamb steaks with salt on both sides, then grill them on each side for a few minutes, just to get some char lines. Set aside.

Drain off the oil from the anchovies and use about 2 teaspoonfuls to coat the base of a flameproof casserole dish or a lidded sauté pan. Finely chop the anchovies.

Heat the oil, then add the onion. Fry briskly for a few minutes, until it starts to brown around the edges. Add the anchovies, garlic and all but a few spikes of rosemary, then pour in the red wine. Season with plenty of pepper. Add the steaks along with about 100ml of water and bring to the boil.

Turn the heat down to a low simmer and leave to cook gently until the lamb is almost tender. Add the cavolo nero on top and leave to steam for a further 15–20 minutes.

While the lamb and cavolo are cooking, make the mash. Put the swede and carrot in a steamer basket with a good pinch of salt and steam over boiling water for 15–20 minutes. Remove from the steamer and mash well. Beat in the mustard and crème fraiche.

Finely chop the remaining rosemary and sprinkle it, together with a squeeze of lemon juice, over the lamb just before serving. The garlic cloves can be lightly mashed into the cooking liquor or left whole. Serve the lamb, onions and cavolo nero with the mash.

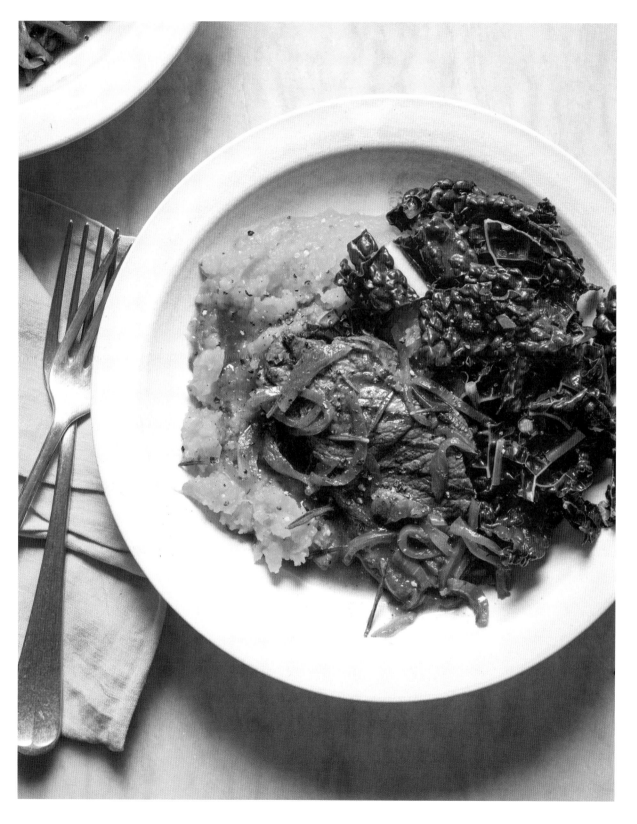

INFO PER SERVING: CALORIES 400   PROTEIN (G) 30   CARBS (G) 27   SUGAR (G) 25   FAT (G) 14
SATURATED FAT (G) 6   FIBRE (G) 14   SALT (G) 0.9

LAMB & RICE SALAD

2 lamb leg steaks
    (about 300g in total)
zest and juice of ½ lemon
1 tsp dried mint
1 tsp sumac (optional)
sea salt and black pepper

Salad
4 apricots, halved and stoned
4 baby leeks or large spring onions
100g asparagus spears
100g broad beans
150g cooked black wild rice
    or red rice (about 60g
    uncooked weight)
200g baby spinach

Dressing
1 tsp olive oil
juice of ½ lemon

Garnish
leaves from a small bunch
    of parsley
leaves from a small bunch of mint
fronds from a small bunch of dill
    (optional)

There's something about the sweetness of lamb that's bang on with a bit of fruit, so we hope you enjoy this colourful and tasty salad. There's loads of great veg to bulk out the meat so you only need a small amount of rice, which keeps the carb content down.

First trim the lamb steaks of any thick pieces of fat. Put the lemon zest and juice in a bowl and add the mint and the sumac, if using. Mix thoroughly. Season the steaks with salt and pepper, then add them to the bowl, making sure they are well coated with the lemon mixture.

Heat a griddle pan. Grill the apricots, leeks or spring onions and the asparagus spears, turning them regularly until softened and lightly charred. Remove from the griddle. Slice the apricots into wedges and cut the asparagus and leeks or spring onions into 3cm lengths. Cook the broad beans in boiling water until tender. Set aside.

Add the steaks to the griddle pan and grill for several minutes on each side until well charred and cooked to your liking but still slightly pink in the middle. Remove from the pan and slice thinly.

Arrange the cooked rice and baby spinach on a large serving dish and top with the asparagus, leeks or spring onions, broad beans, most of the herbs and the slices of lamb. Toss lightly, then add the apricots.

Whisk the olive oil and lemon juice together with salt and pepper. Drizzle over the salad and garnish with the remaining herbs. Serve while the meat and vegetables are still warm.

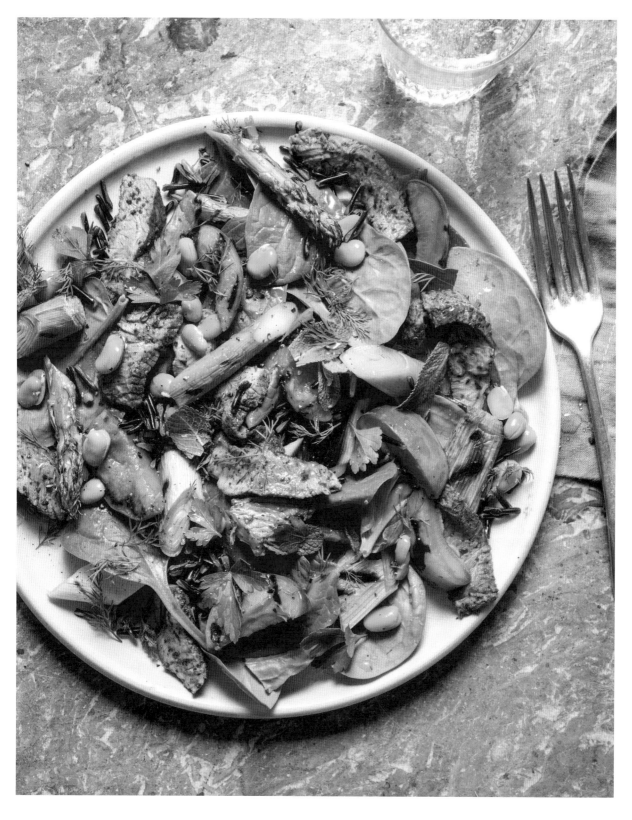

INFO PER SERVING: CALORIES 328   PROTEIN (G) 25   CARBS (G) 34   SUGAR (G) 5   FAT (G) 8
SATURATED FAT (G) 3   FIBRE (G) 8   SALT (G) TRACE

PORK & KIMCHI FRIED RICE

2 tsp vegetable oil

bunch of spring onions, whites and greens separated, sliced into rounds

15g root ginger, finely chopped

3 garlic cloves, finely chopped

200g lean pork mince

200g drained kimchi, finely chopped (reserve 50ml of the liquid)

400g cooked brown rice (125g uncooked)

250g cavolo nero, shredded and blanched

100g frozen peas, defrosted

a few drops sesame oil (optional)

small bunch of coriander, chopped

1 tsp sesame seeds (preferably black)

sea salt and black pepper

Sauce

1 tbsp dark soy sauce

1–3 tsp gochujang (or to taste, optional)

50ml kimchi juice

Optional extra

4 fried eggs

This is a cracking little recipe and so easy. You don't need a lot of pork, so the dish is not high in fat, but the meat adds loads of flavour and goes brilliantly with the kimchi. Gochujang is a Korean fermented paste that's available in most supermarkets now. We've made it optional but it's well worth including, as it adds a great punch of flavour. Both kimchi and gochujang are fermented foods and we know that they are good for the gut – as well as being dead tasty. You can buy good kimchi in the shops now, but if you do want to make your own, have a look at our recipe on page 176.

First make the sauce. Whisk together the soy sauce with the gochujang chilli paste, if using, and the kimchi juice. Set aside.

Heat the oil in a wok and add the white spring onion rounds, ginger, garlic and pork mince. Season with salt and pepper. Stir-fry until the pork is well browned, then stir in the kimchi. Cook for another couple of minutes, then stir in the rice, cavolo nero and peas. Pour in the sauce and continue to cook, turning everything over until it is all piping hot.

Drizzle over a few drops of sesame oil, if using, then garnish with the coriander, spring onion greens and sesame seeds. Serve with a fried egg on top if you fancy.

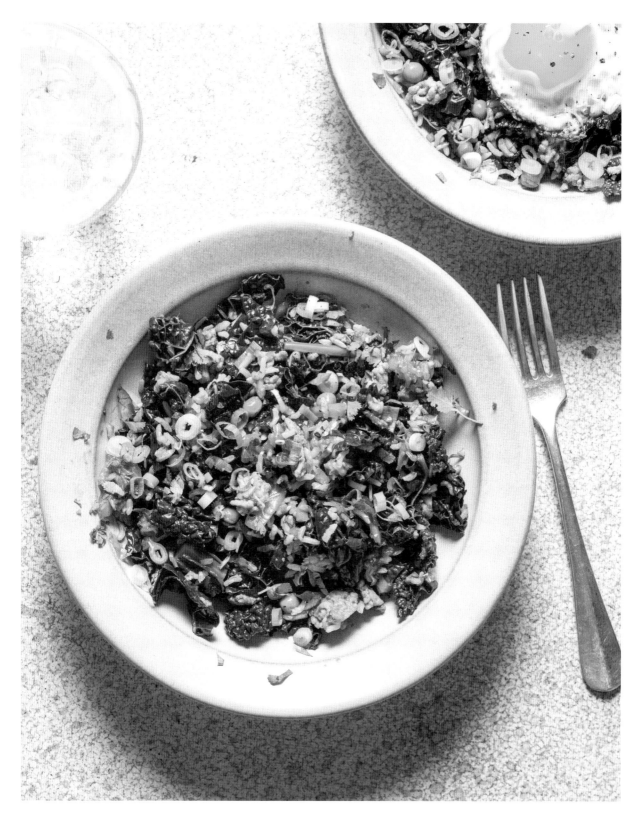

INFO PER SERVING/WITH EGG: CALORIES 217/337   PROTEIN (G) 18/27   CARBS (G) 16.5/16.5
SUGAR (G) 4/4   FAT (G) 7.5/17   SATURATED FAT (G) 2/4   FIBRE (G) 5/5   SALT (G) 0.9/1.2

BRAISED AUBERGINES WITH PORK

2 tsp vegetable oil
1 large aubergine, diced
100g lean minced pork
15g root ginger, finely chopped
3 garlic cloves, finely chopped
2 red chillies, finely chopped
½ tsp Szechuan peppercorns, crushed
½ tsp Chinese five-spice powder
200g shiitake mushrooms, sliced or halved
200g kale, shredded, or kalettes, halved
sea salt and black pepper

Sauce
150ml vegetable or chicken stock
2 tbsp soy sauce
1 tbsp rice wine vinegar

To serve
drizzle of sesame oil
2 spring onions, finely chopped
brown rice or noodles (optional)

You're going to love this Chinese-inspired aubergine dish, spiced up with chillies and Szechuan peppercorns. It makes a nice low-carb supper for two or you could add rice or noodles and serve four. Don't forget to add the extra calories for the carbs though, if you're counting.

Heat the oil in a wok. When it is smoking, add the diced aubergine and quickly brown it all over. Add the pork, ginger, garlic, chillies, peppercorns, Chinese five-spice and mushrooms, and continue to stir-fry until the pork is just cooked through. Season with salt and pepper and stir in the greens.

Mix the sauce ingredients together and pour the mixture over the contents of the wok. Stir to combine, then turn down the heat a little and cover the pan. Leave to simmer until the aubergines and greens are completely cooked through – this will take about 10 minutes.

Serve with a drizzle of sesame oil and the spring onions. Add some rice or noodles if you like.

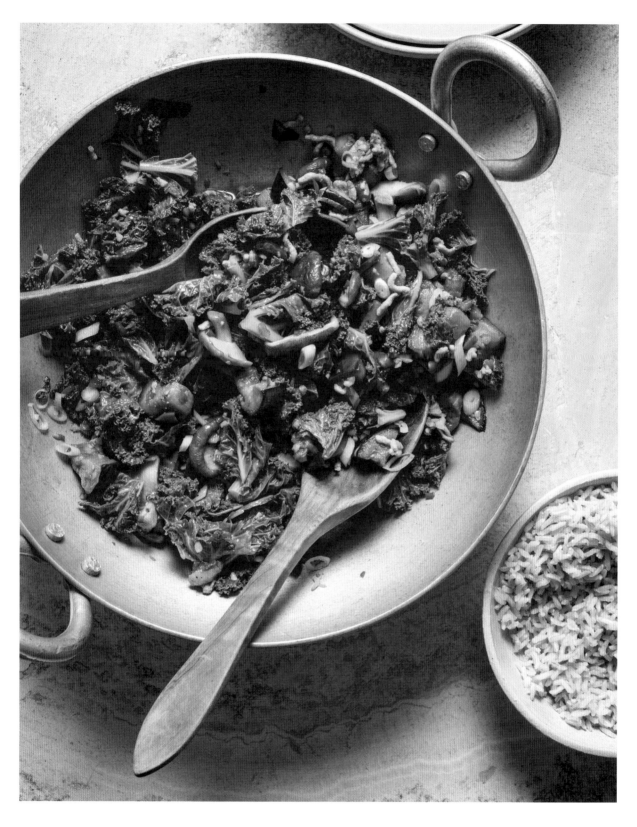

INFO PER SERVING: CALORIES 253   PROTEIN (G) 20   CARBS (G) 15   SUGAR (G) 9   FAT (G) 10
SATURATED FAT (G) 2   FIBRE (G) 11   SALT (G) 2.4

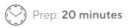
PORK & LENTIL RISSOLES

250g pork mince or 200g cooked
   pork, finely diced
2 tsp olive oil
1 small fennel bulb, very finely
   chopped, any fronds reserved
2 garlic cloves, finely chopped
zest of 1 lemon
leaves from a large sprig of thyme
   or 1 tsp dried thyme
250g cooked brown lentils
   (from a can)
50g breadcrumbs
1 egg
sea salt and black pepper

Sauce
1 tsp olive oil
1 onion, very finely chopped
2 red peppers, finely chopped
3 garlic cloves, finely chopped
1 tsp fennel seeds
1 tsp smoked paprika
400g can of tomatoes
leaves from a small bunch
   of parsley, finely chopped

Rissoles seem to have gone a bit out of fashion, but we reckon they are well worth reviving and the lentils here help a little meat go a long way. Our recipe uses leftover cooked pork or mince, but it will work with lamb too. Some greens on the side would be good and perhaps some celeriac mash (see page 169) to soak up the rich sauce. The lentils need to be quite soft to blend well with the other ingredients, so the ones in a can rather than a pouch are probably best.

First make the rissoles. If using the pork mince, put it in a heated frying pan and cook until well browned. Drain and set to one side.

Heat the olive oil in a frying pan and add the fennel. Cook over a medium heat, stirring regularly, until the fennel is soft and translucent. Add the garlic and cook for a further couple of minutes. Remove from the heat and tip into a bowl, then stir in the lemon zest, thyme, lentils, breadcrumbs and the browned mince or diced pork. Season well with salt and pepper, then stir in the egg. Mix thoroughly (kneading with your hands works best), until the mixture clumps well together.

Preheat the oven to 180°C/Fan 160°C /Gas 4. Divide the mixture into 8, shape into patties and place them on a lined baking tray. Bake in the preheated oven for 20 minutes, until firm and lightly browned.

To make the sauce, heat the olive oil in a wide pan with a lid. Add the onion and peppers, fry over a medium heat for a few minutes, then add the garlic and fennel seeds. Add a splash of water, season with salt and pepper, then cover the pan. Leave to sweat gently for a few more minutes until the onion and peppers are tender.

Stir in the paprika and tomatoes, then swill out the can with 200ml of water and add this to the pan. Bring to the boil, then turn the heat down, cover the pan and leave the sauce to simmer for 10 minutes. Remove the lid and simmer for another 5 minutes.

Add the rissoles to the pan and simmer gently for 5 minutes. Sprinkle with the parsley and any reserved fronds of fennel and serve.

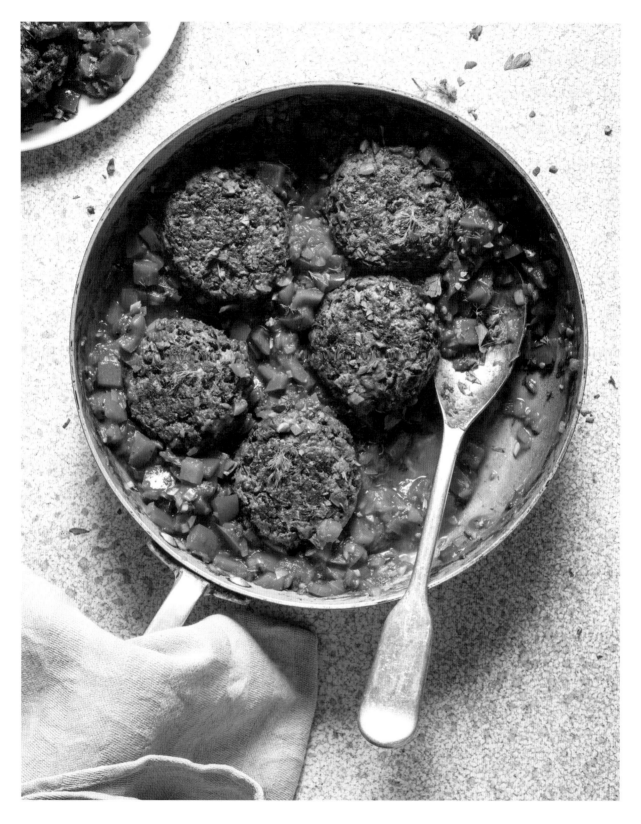

INFO PER SERVING: CALORIES 305   PROTEIN (G) 21.5   CARBS (G) 26   SUGAR (G) 10   FAT (G) 11
SATURATED FAT (G) 3   FIBRE (G) 7   SALT (G) TRACE

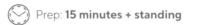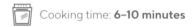
STEAK & CANNELLINI BEAN SALAD

500g bavette steak
1 tsp dried oregano
sea salt and black pepper

Salad
100g rocket leaves
1 red onion, finely sliced and
    soaked in cold, salted water
    for 30 minutes
2 tomatoes, diced
400g can of cannellini beans,
    drained
1 tsp olive oil
small bunch of parsley, finely
    chopped
6 caper berries, stems removed,
    sliced into rounds
leaves from a few sprigs of fresh
    oregano (optional)

Dressing
1 tsp olive oil
1 tbsp sherry vinegar
zest and juice of ½ orange
pinch of chilli flakes

Bavette steak is also known as flank steak and is cheaper than some cuts. We love it for its flavour but take care not to overcook it or it will be tough. If you're feeling flush, you could use sirloin instead. Caper berries are the fruits of the caper plant and are usually sold on the stems. They're bigger than capers, which are actually the pickled flower buds, and they have a milder flavour that's just right in this salad.

Remove the steak from the fridge an hour before you want to cook it, so it can come up to room temperature. Season it with plenty of salt and pepper and sprinkle with the oregano.

Heat a large griddle pan until it is too hot to hold your hand over, then add the steak. Leave it without turning for several minutes until it lifts off the griddle cleanly and has deep char lines. Cook the other side for several minutes, again until it will lift off cleanly. This will give you a steak between rare and medium rare depending on how thick it is. Cook for another 2–3 minutes on each side for medium rare to medium. Place it on a chopping board and leave to rest. Drain all the juices into a bowl and thinly slice the meat.

Add the dressing ingredients to the bowl containing the meat juices and season. Taste and adjust accordingly, adding a little more vinegar if necessary.

Put the rocket, drained onion and tomatoes in a bowl. Toss the beans with the olive oil, parsley leaves and caper berries and season with salt and pepper. Add these to the other salad ingredients, then add the slices of beef. Pour over the dressing and toss to combine. Garnish with the oregano leaves, if using.

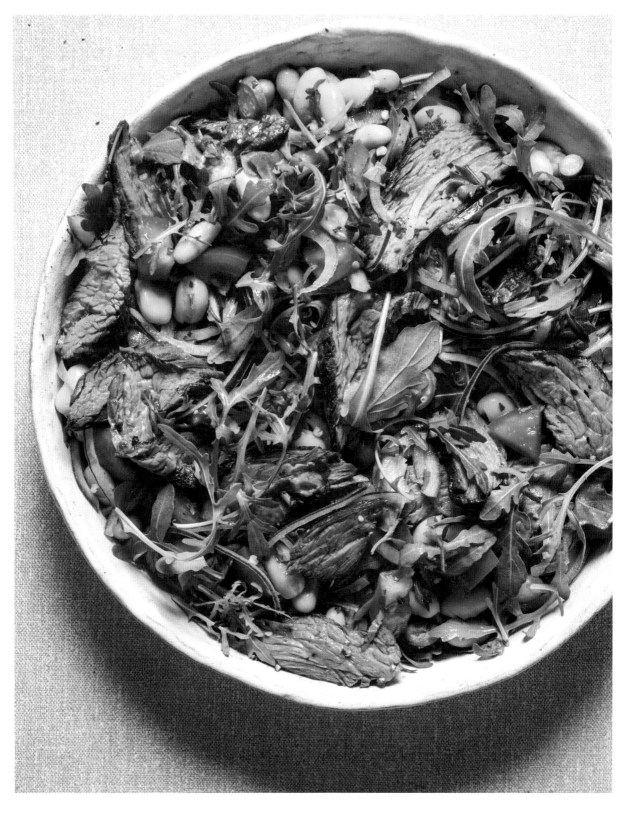

INFO PER SERVING:　CALORIES 332　PROTEIN (G) 30　CARBS (G) 15.5　SUGAR (G) 5　FAT (G) 15
SATURATED FAT (G) 6　FIBRE (G) 6.5　SALT (G) TRACE

SLOW-COOKED FEATHERBLADE

1 tbsp olive oil
1 large onion, sliced
2 carrots, thickly sliced
2 celery sticks, sliced
600g featherblade steak (or any braising/casserole steak), diced
10g dried mushrooms, soaked in warm water (optional)
½ bulb of garlic, broken up into unpeeled cloves
1 bouquet garni made up of parsley, bay leaves and thyme
500ml beef or mushroom stock
1 tsp wholegrain mustard
sea salt and black pepper

Featherblade is ideally suited to slow, gentle cooking, as in this proper tasty braised dish. The sauce is thickened by pushing the vegetables through a sieve back into the cooking liquid, so you don't need any flour or other thickening agent. The result is amazingly flavourful but very little trouble to make – the oven does most of the work. Nice with some green veg and mash for a supper that's a real winter warmer – you'll find some good mash recipes in the last chapter of this book.

Preheat the oven to 160°C/Fan 140°C/Gas 3.

Heat the olive oil in a large flameproof casserole dish. Add the onion, carrots and celery and fry them over a high heat until they're starting to take on some colour, then push them to one side. Season the steak with salt and pepper and add it to the casserole. Sear on all sides.

Drain the mushrooms, if using, and chop them finely. Add them and the strained soaking liquor to the dish, then add the garlic, bouquet garni and stock. Bring to the boil, then cover the dish and transfer it to the oven. Cook in the preheated oven for 2–3 hours until the beef is very tender, checking from 2 hours onwards.

Remove the casserole dish from the oven. Transfer the beef to a plate, discard the bouquet garni and push the remaining contents – liquid and vegetables – through a coarse sieve. Pour the liquid back into the casserole dish and stir in the mustard. Put the beef back in the casserole and heat it through before serving. This is nice with some mash and greens.

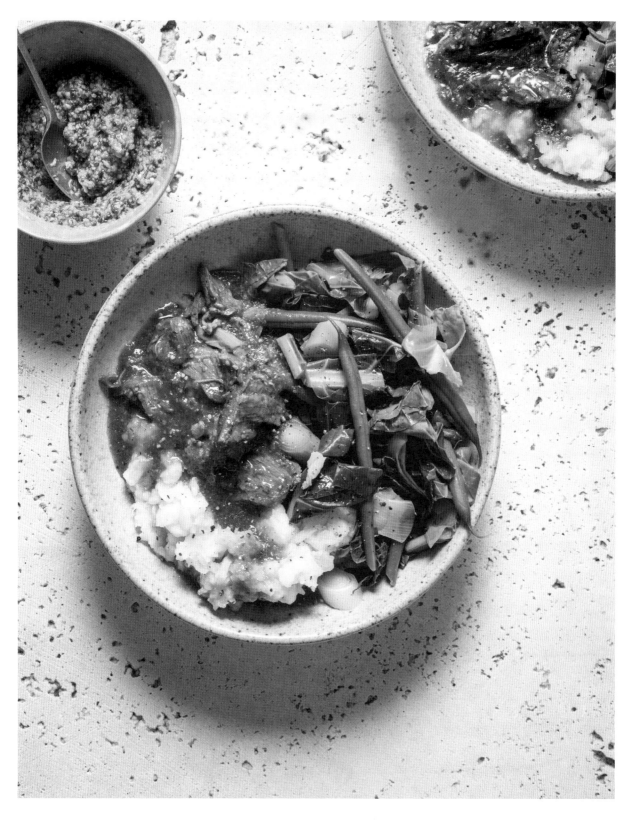

INFO PER SERVING (WITHOUT MASH OR GREENS):   CALORIES 263   PROTEIN (G) 34   CARBS (G) 8
SUGAR (G) 7   FAT (G) 10   SATURATED FAT (G) 3   FIBRE (G) 4   SALT (G) 1.1

BOILED BEEF WITH CARROTS & BEETROOT

1kg silverside or topside, any
   added fat removed

2 celery sticks, coarsely chopped

12 chantenay carrots, trimmed
   (or 4 carrots cut into chunks)

250g raw beetroots, peeled and
   cut into wedges

1 onion, thickly sliced

1 bouquet garni made up of 1 tsp
   caraway seeds, 1 tsp juniper
   berries, 2 cloves and 2 bay
   leaves, tied in a muslin bag

2 tbsp tomato purée

1 litre beef stock

sea salt and black pepper

Dumplings (optional)

150g self-raising flour

75g plain yoghurt

1 egg

3 tbsp finely chopped dill
   or parsley

1 tsp mustard or horseradish
   sauce (optional)

Boiled beef and carrots is a much-loved traditional dish and we like to dial it up by adding beetroot, which goes so well with beef. It's rich in nutrients too and low in calories. If your beef is covered in a layer of fat, make sure you remove this before cooking. The fat is needed for roasting the meat in the oven, but not when pot-roasting like this. Add dumplings if you like – these are surprisingly light.

If the beef has been rolled and tied with an extra covering of fat, untie it, remove the fat and tie it up again.

Season the beef, then put it in a large pan or a flameproof casserole dish with the vegetables and the bouquet garni. Whisk the tomato purée with the beef stock and pour the mixture over the contents of the pan. Add water until the beef is just covered.

Bring the water to the boil, then turn down the heat and cover the pan. Leave to simmer very gently, turning the meat over every so often, until it's tender. This will take about 2 hours.

If you want to add the dumplings, put the flour in a bowl and add salt and pepper. Add the yoghurt, egg, herbs – and the mustard or horseradish if you want your dumplings to have a kick. Mix thoroughly to make a fairly dense, sticky dough.

Make sure the liquid in the pan is at least at simmering point, then drop heaped dessertspoons of the dough on top of the meat and vegetables, spacing them out well. You should get 8 dumplings. Cover and leave to cook for another 15 minutes. The dumplings will be well risen – almost puffed up – and with a set, glossy looking top.

Transfer the meat to a board and slice it coarsely. Remove the bouquet garni and discard it. Serve the beef in shallow bowls with the vegetables and some of the cooking liquid ladled over the top, plus the dumplings, if including.

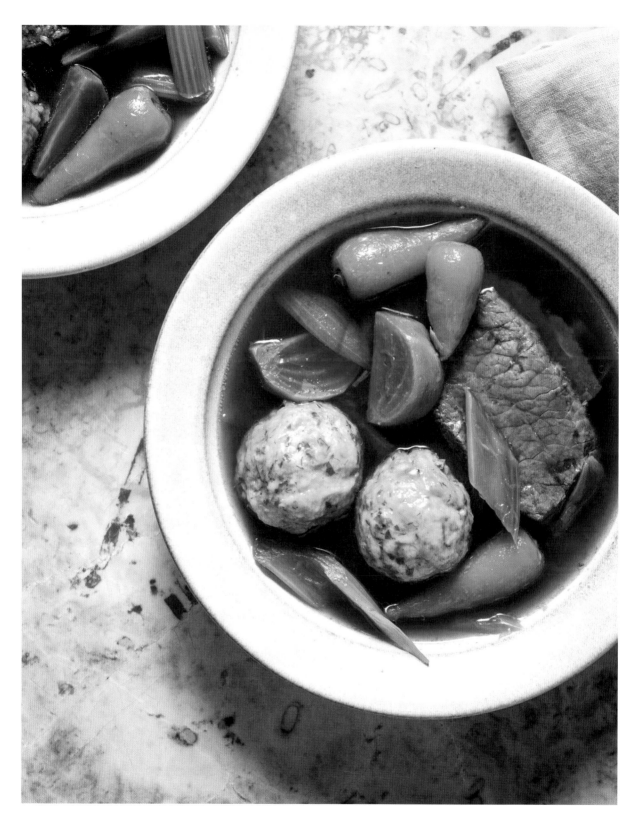

INFO PER SERVING/WITH DUMPLINGS: CALORIES 395/568   PROTEIN (G) 63/70   CARBS (G) 14.5/45
SUGAR (G) 13.5/15   FAT (G) 8/10.5   SATURATED FAT 3/4   FIBRE (G) 7/8   SALT (G) 2/2.5

MEATBALLS WITH CHIP SHOP CURRY SAUCE

Meatballs
400g lean minced beef
1 small onion, grated
1 medium carrot, grated
2 garlic cloves, crushed
2 tbsp finely chopped coriander stems
1 tsp curry powder
25g breadcrumbs
25g thick yoghurt or kefir
chopped coriander, to garnish
sea salt and black pepper

Sauce
1 tsp coconut oil
2 large onions, finely sliced
1 carrot, finely sliced
4 garlic cloves, finely sliced
15g root ginger, finely chopped
1 apple, peeled and chopped
25g raisins
2 tbsp mild curry powder
½–1 tsp cayenne, to taste
1 tbsp tomato purée
500ml chicken or vegetable stock
1 tsp Worcestershire sauce
1 tsp apple cider vinegar
squeeze of lemon juice

We like to have something a bit naughty now and then and a good chip shop curry sauce brings back happy memories of many a feast. It works a treat with these spicy meatballs. There are quite a few ingredients here, but they all play a part in the great flavour and the sauce is easy to put together. Serve the meatballs in the sauce as suggested or keep them separate and serve the sauce in bowls for dipping.

Preheat the oven to 200°C/Fan 180°C/Gas 6 and line a baking tray with parchment.

Put all the ingredients for the meatballs in a bowl with plenty of seasoning and mix thoroughly. Divide the mixture into 20 balls, then place them on the baking tray and bake for 15 minutes.

To make the sauce, melt the coconut oil in a pan, then add the onions and carrot. Add a splash of water, stir to coat, then cover and leave to cook over a medium-high heat. Cook, stirring regularly, for about 10 minutes until the vegetables are softened and starting to brown.

Turn up the heat and add the garlic, ginger, apple and raisins. Stir for a couple of minutes, then add the curry powder, cayenne and tomato purée. Stir so a paste forms around the vegetables and fruit, then pour in the stock. Stir to deglaze the base of the pan, then add the Worcestershire sauce and vinegar. Season with salt and pepper. Bring to the boil, then cover, reduce the heat and simmer for 20 minutes. Blitz in a blender or food processor until smooth. Taste and add a squeeze of lemon juice and more chilli if necessary.

Add the meatballs to the sauce and simmer for a few minutes, then garnish with some chopped coriander and serve.

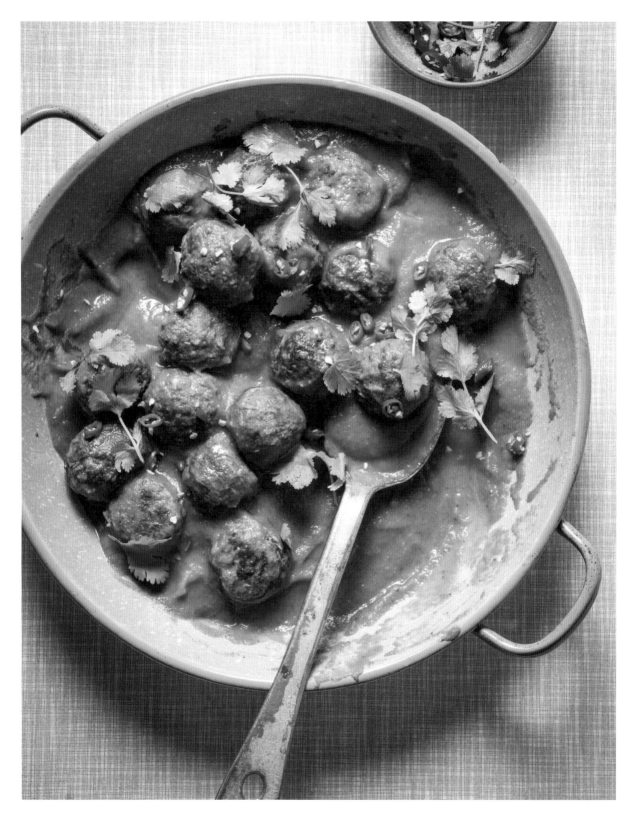

INFO PER SERVING: CALORIES 361   PROTEIN (G) 29   CARBS (G) 28   SUGAR (G) 19   FAT (G) 13
SATURATED FAT (G) 5   FIBRE (G) 8   SALT (G) 0.7

A TOU
SWEE

COCONUT RICE PUDDING WITH PASSION FRUIT

75g short-grain pudding rice
750ml coconut milk
   (not from a can)
1 cinnamon stick
2 cardamom pods
strip of pared lime zest (optional)
25ml maple syrup
pinch of sea salt
2 large passion fruit

The secret to success here is to use the pouring coconut milk that's sold in bottles or cartons, rather than the stuff in cans. The pouring coconut milk is blended with rice and has a fraction of the calories of full-fat coconut milk and less than the reduced-fat coconut milk in a can. The other benefit of using the pouring coconut milk is that it doesn't separate. This version of rice pudding is easy to make, not high in calories or fat and completely delicious. It's also great with slices of fresh mango on the top instead of passion fruit.

To make the rice pudding, put the rice in a saucepan with the milk, spices, lime zest, if using, and the maple syrup. Add a pinch of salt and slowly bring to the boil, stirring regularly. Turn down the heat and cook gently for about half an hour, until the rice has swelled up and thickened and is tender.

Remove the pan from the heat and allow the rice to cool a little. Fish out the cinnamon stick, lime zest and cardamom pods before serving.

Cut the passion fruit in half and spoon the pulp and seeds over the servings of rice pudding.

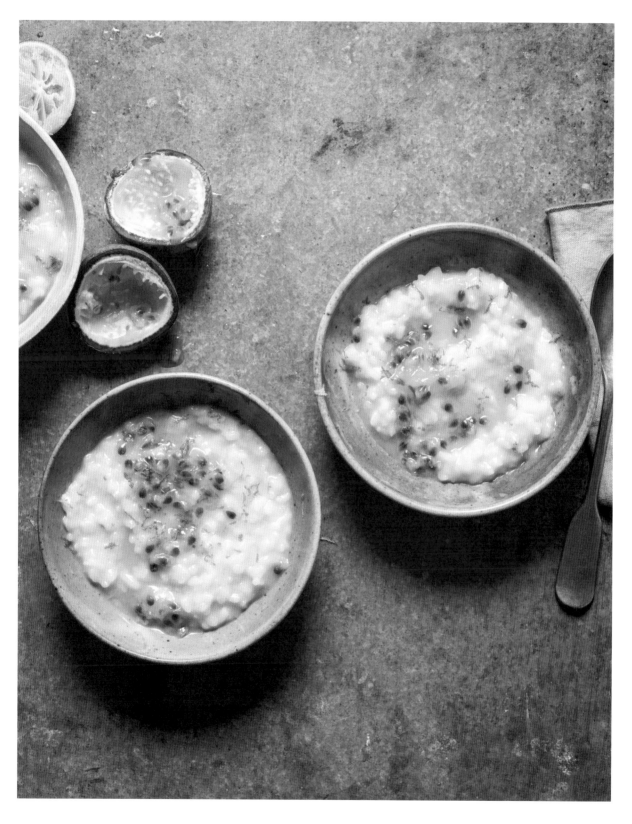

INFO PER SERVING: CALORIES 124   PROTEIN (G) 1.5   CARBS (G) 25   SUGAR (G) 8   FAT (G) 2
SATURATED FAT (G) 2   FIBRE (G) 0.5   SALT (G) 0.5

HONEY & BUTTERMILK PANNA COTTA

2 gelatine leaves
150ml whole milk
100ml single cream
50g honey
oil, for greasing
½ tsp vanilla extract
150ml buttermilk

To serve
seasonal berries

Who would have thought you could make a healthy panna cotta? Always a popular pud, it's easy to make and great when you've got friends coming round, as it can be prepared well in advance and left to chill. This version is light and smooth, with a beautiful flavour of honey and vanilla. Just be careful with the gelatine. Two leaves worked well with the brand we had, but check the packet and make sure you're using the right quantity of gelatine for the amount of liquid.

Cover the gelatine leaves in cold water and leave them to soak for a few minutes, until very pliable.

Put the milk, cream and honey in a small saucepan and heat, whisking constantly, until well combined. Wring out the gelatine leaves and add them to the pan. Stir until the gelatine has dissolved, then strain the mixture through a fine sieve into a jug.

Lightly oil 4 ramekin dishes.

Add the vanilla extract and the buttermilk to the jug. Stir to combine, then pour the mixture into the prepared ramekins. Leave to cool, then transfer to the fridge and leave to chill until set – this will take about 3 hours. Serve with berries.

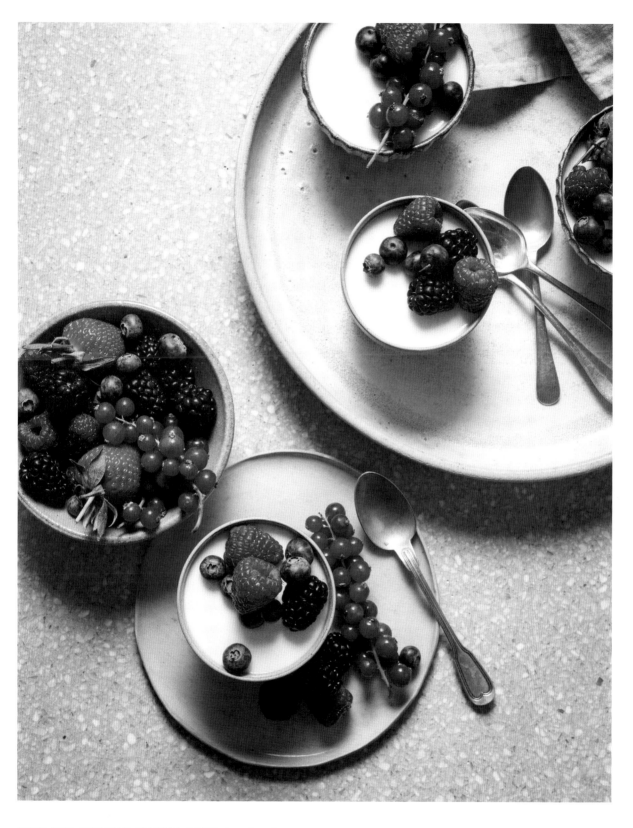

INFO PER SERVING (PANNA COTTA): CALORIES 124 PROTEIN (G) 4 CARBS (G) 13 SUGAR (G) 13
FAT (G) 6.5 SATURATED FAT (G) 4 FIBRE (G) 0 SALT (G) TRACE

MOJITO FRUIT SALAD

4 kiwi fruit, peeled and diced
150g green grapes, halved
300g green-fleshed melon,
   peeled and diced
100g cucumber, peeled and diced
small mint leaves, to garnish

Dressing
zest and juice of 1 lime
1 tbsp sugar or xylitol
about 25 small mint leaves

To serve (optional)
1–3 tsp rum (per person)
pinch of salt
pinch of chilli powder

One for the cocktail lovers out there! Wow – we love this simple fruity dessert. It's low in calories and very low in fat but with a banging flavour. Obviously, it's excellent with the rum, but if you're making it for kids or non-drinkers it's still mega delicious and refreshing without. Try it with the chilli too – it works really well. Making the salad with xylitol (a natural alternative to sugar) reduces the calorie count slightly and the lime and mint is so intense you won't notice any difference in taste.

Put all the fruit and the cucumber in a bowl and chill well.

When you are almost ready to serve, put the lime zest and juice, sugar or xylitol and mint leaves in a bowl and muddle them together (smash them about a bit) until the mint has broken down and most of the sugar or xylitol has dissolved. Pour this over the fruit and mix well.

Divide the fruit between bowls and add the mint leaves as a garnish. Add rum, salt and/or chilli as you like.

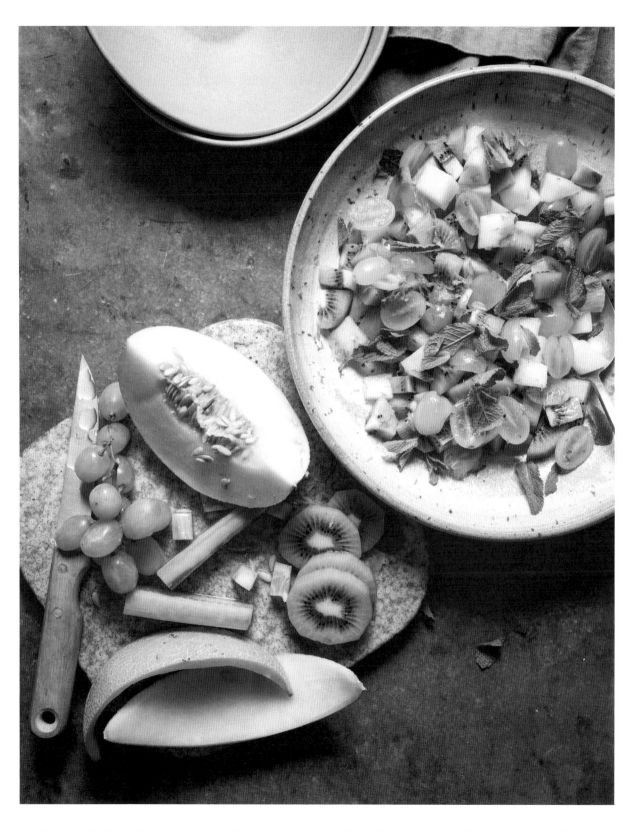

INFO PER SERVING WITH SUGAR/WITH XYLITOL: CALORIES 97/82 PROTEIN (G) 1.5/1.5 CARBS (G) 20/16
SUGAR (G) 20/16   FAT (G) 0.5/0.5   SATURATED FAT (G) 0/0 FIBRE (G) 3/3   SALT (G) TRACE/TRACE

Serves: **4**   Prep: **10 minutes**   Cooking time: **30–35 minutes**

CRUNCHY APPLE CRUMBLE

1 cooking apple, peeled, cored
   and chopped
3 eating apples, peeled, cored
   and chopped
25g raisins
1 tsp cinnamon
1 tbsp honey or maple syrup

Topping
50g wholemeal flour
50g butter, chilled and diced
25g porridge oats
25g flax seeds
½ tsp cinnamon
2 tbsp maple syrup

It's nice to have a treat once in a while, even when you're watching your weight, and we do love a crumble. This version contains less sugar and butter than the usual recipe but it's still lip-smackingly good, and the oats and seeds make it nice and crunchy. Using a mix of cooking and eating apples really helps, as the eating apples are sweet, so need less sugar, and the cooking apples provide a tartness that's bang on.

Preheat the oven to 180°C/Fan 160°C/Gas 4.

Put all the apples in an ovenproof dish and stir in the raisins and cinnamon. Drizzle over the honey or maple syrup and mix thoroughly.

Put the flour into a bowl, add the butter and rub it in with your fingers. Stir in the porridge oats, flax seeds and cinnamon and mix well, then drizzle over the maple syrup and mix again.

Sprinkle the mixture over the apples in a thin, even layer. Put the dish on a baking tray and bake in the preheated oven for 30–35 minutes until lightly browned. Serve with crème fraiche if you like.

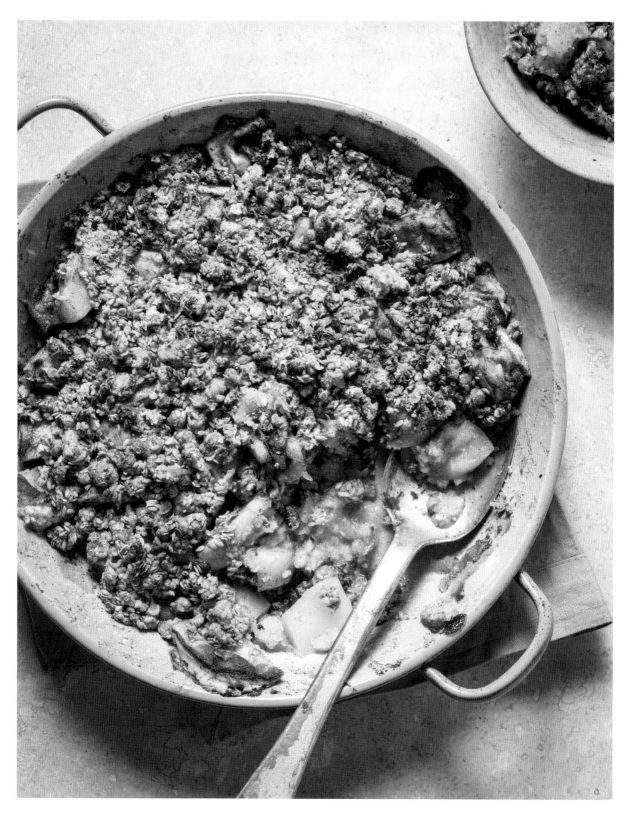

INFO PER SERVING: CALORIES 331 PROTEIN (G) 4.5 CARBS (G) 43 SUGAR (G) 20.5 FAT (G) 14
SATURATED FAT (G) 7 FIBRE (G) 5.5 SALT (G) TRACE

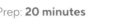
CARROT CAKE

butter, for greasing
200g wholemeal flour
2 tsp baking powder
½ tsp bicarbonate of soda
½ tsp ground cardamom
pinch of salt
100g light soft brown sugar
50ml maple syrup
zest of 1 orange
3 eggs
75ml sunflower or rapeseed oil
50g plain yoghurt
50g walnuts or pecans, chopped
200g carrots, grated
150g raisins

Icing (optional)
50g quark
50g cream cheese
25g thick plain yoghurt
25g icing sugar
a few drops of vanilla extract

Not a dish for every day but we have reduced the calories in this cake by cutting back on the sugar and oil, so you can have your cake and eat it – occasionally at least! Adding yoghurt helps keep the cake moist. If you like, you could replace the sugar with xylitol (a natural alternative to sugar) to reduce the calories still further. Icing is optional but if you do add icing, keep the cake in the fridge, as there isn't a high enough sugar content to preserve the dairy safely.

Preheat the oven to 180°C/Fan 160°C/Gas 4. Butter a 20cm round cake tin and line it with baking parchment.

Mix the flour, baking powder, bicarb and cardamom with a generous pinch of salt. In a separate bowl, beat together the sugar, maple syrup, orange zest, eggs and oil until well combined. Fold in the flour mixture followed by the yoghurt to make a smooth batter, then stir in the nuts, grated carrots and raisins.

Scrape the mixture into the prepared tin and bake in the oven for about 45 minutes until well risen, springy to the touch and slightly shrunken away from the sides. Remove from the oven and leave the cake in the tin for 10 minutes before turning it out on to a cooling rack.

To make the icing, if using, beat together all the ingredients until thick and smooth. When the cake is completely cool, spread the icing over the top with a palette knife. If not serving immediately, store the cake in an airtight container in the fridge.

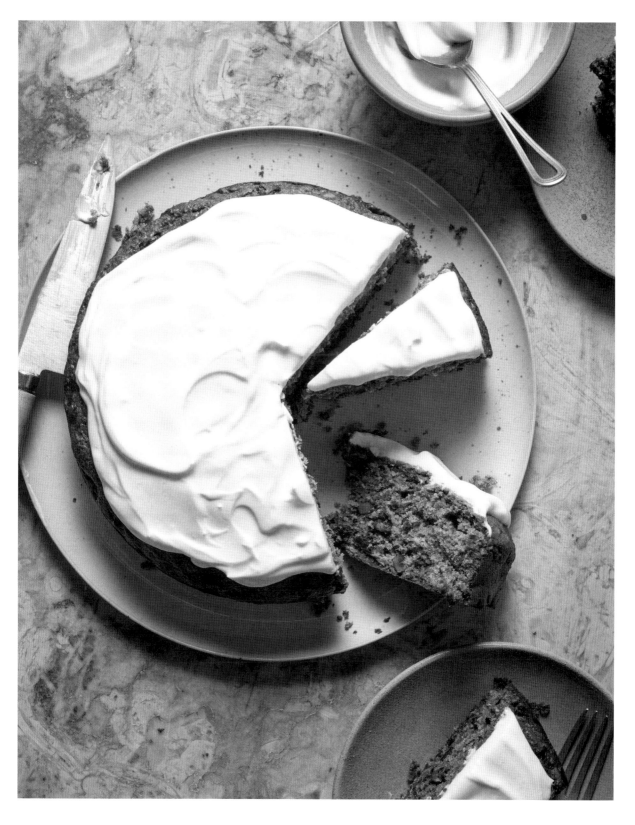

INFO PER SLICE WITHOUT ICING/WITH ICING: CALORIES 358/392   PROTEIN (G) 8/9   CARBS (G) 48/51
SUGAR (G) 30/34   FAT (G) 14/15.5   SATURATED FAT (G) 2/3   FIBRE (G) 4/4   SALT (G) 0.8/0.8

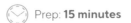
RASPBERRY & ROSE FAIRY CAKES

125g plain flour
1 tsp baking powder
pinch of salt
50g butter, softened
75g caster sugar
2 eggs
1–2 tbsp milk
50g raspberries, lightly crushed,
    plus extra to garnish

Glaze (optional)
50g icing sugar
a few drops of rose water
1–3 tsp milk

These are classy little numbers for teatime and just one with your cuppa won't upset your waistline too much. Make sure not to over mix the raspberries in the cake batter or it will go grey, not a pleasing pink!

Preheat the oven to 180°C/Fan 160°C/Gas 4. Line a 12-hole fairy cake tin with paper cases.

Mix the plain flour and baking powder with a pinch of salt. Beat the butter and sugar together with electric hand beaters or in a stand mixer until fluffy.

Beat in the eggs and flour, followed by the milk, a tablespoon at a time, to make a mixture with a dropping consistency. Gently fold in the raspberries but don't stir too much. Aim for a ripple effect not a pink sponge.

Spoon the batter into the fairy cake cases – they will take roughly 1 heaped tablespoon of mixture each. Bake in the oven for 12–15 minutes until the cakes are well risen, light golden brown in colour and springy to the touch.

To make the glaze, if using, sieve the icing sugar into a bowl, then whisk in the rose water and the milk, a little at a time until you have a thick icing. Be sparing with the milk as the icing will become very runny quickly.

When the fairy cakes are completely cool, swirl a little of the icing on the top of each one – about 1 teaspoonful per cake – and top with an extra raspberry. Alternatively, just dust the cakes with icing sugar.

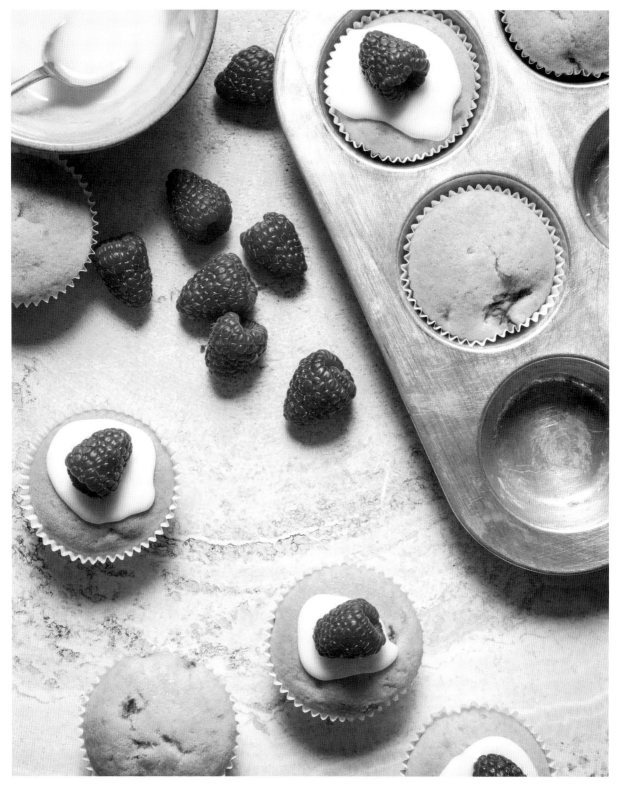

INFO PER CAKE/WITH GLAZE: CALORIES 109/127   PROTEIN (G) 2/2.5   CARBS (G) 14.5/19
SUGAR (G) 6.5/11   FAT (G) 4.5/4.5   SATURATED FAT (G) 2.5/2.5   FIBRE (G) 0.5/0.5
SALT (G) TRACE/TRACE

CUSTARD TARTLETS

8 thin slices of white bread, crusts removed
1 large egg, beaten
5g butter
60ml crème fraiche
1 tbsp maple syrup
zest of 1 clementine or mandarin
about 24 small blueberries

Though we say it ourselves, this is a clever way of making some guilt-free custard tarts. One of these goes down a treat with your morning coffee. They look pretty too, as the custard sets around the blueberries nicely, but if you prefer, you could use a teaspoon of jam in each tart instead of the berries. Do follow our method of buttering the warm tin, as it enables you to use very little butter.

Preheat the oven to 200°C/Fan 180°C/Gas 6.

Take each slice of bread and roll it out as flat as you can. Cut out 8 rounds, using a 7.5cm cutter – these should fit the holes in a fairy cake tin perfectly. Press each round firmly into 8 of the holes.

Brush the inside of the bread cases very sparingly with a little of the beaten egg, then put them in the oven for 10 minutes to crisp up. Remove the bread cases from the tin and divide the butter between the 8 holes you are using – the heat should melt the butter immediately so you can brush it round the sides. Return the bread cases to the greased holes in the tin.

Beat the rest of the egg with the crème fraiche, maple syrup and citrus zest. Drop a few berries into each bread case and top with the custard mix. Grate over a little more citrus zest, if you like.

Bake in the oven for 10–12 minutes until the custard has just set and is starting to turn lightly brown.

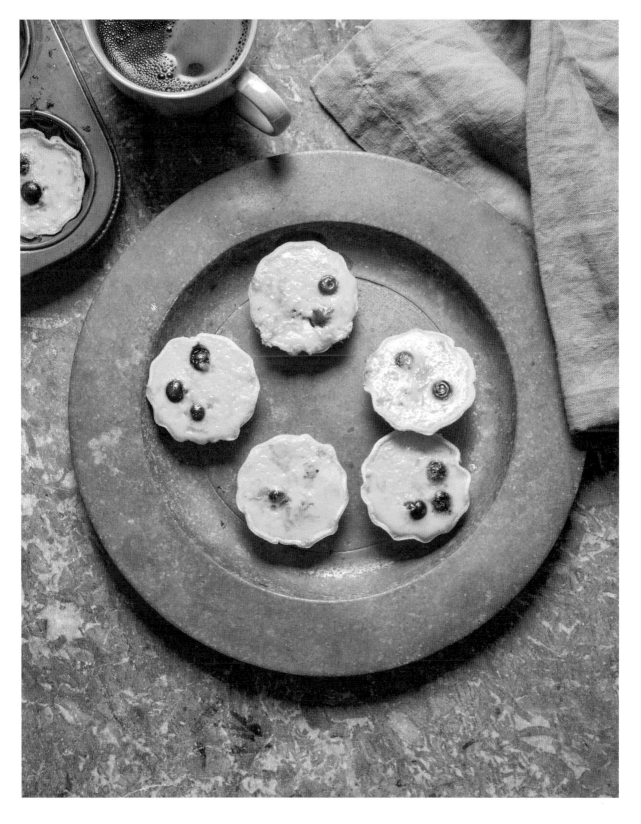

INFO PER TARTLET: CALORIES 118 PROTEIN (G) 3.5 CARBS (G) 14.5 SUGAR (G) 3.5 FAT (G) 5
SATURATED FAT (G) 2.5 FIBRE (G) 1 SALT (G) TRACE

BAKED APPLES WITH DATES & GINGER

4 Bramley apples

8 large soft medjool dates, stones removed, finely chopped

2 pieces of stem ginger, finely chopped

1 tbsp maple syrup

1 tbsp ginger wine (optional)

pinch of cloves

10g butter

To serve (optional)

crème fraiche or yoghurt

An oldie and always a goodie, a baked apple is something we both loved as children and still do. Here, we've given this old favourite a modern twist with a stuffing of dates, ginger and a little syrup, instead of sugar and loads of butter, and we love them as much as ever.

Preheat the oven to 220°C/Fan 200°C/Gas 7.

Prepare the apples. Using an apple corer or a small sharp paring knife, bore a hole from the top through almost to the base, about 2.5–3cm in diameter. Scoop out any seeds but make sure that the base is completely intact. Score a horizontal line around the apples – this will help prevent them from bursting in the oven.

Mix the dates, stem ginger, maple syrup and ginger wine, if using, together with the pinch of cloves. The mixture will have a consistency of a loose purée. Divide this between the apples, stuffing it into each hole and allowing it to dome slightly on top. Then divide the butter between the 4 apples, placing it on top of the piled-up stuffing.

Place the apples in an ovenproof dish. Ideally, they should fit fairly snugly, with a little space around each apple. Bake for about 20 minutes until the apples are tender.

Serve on their own or with some crème fraiche or yoghurt.

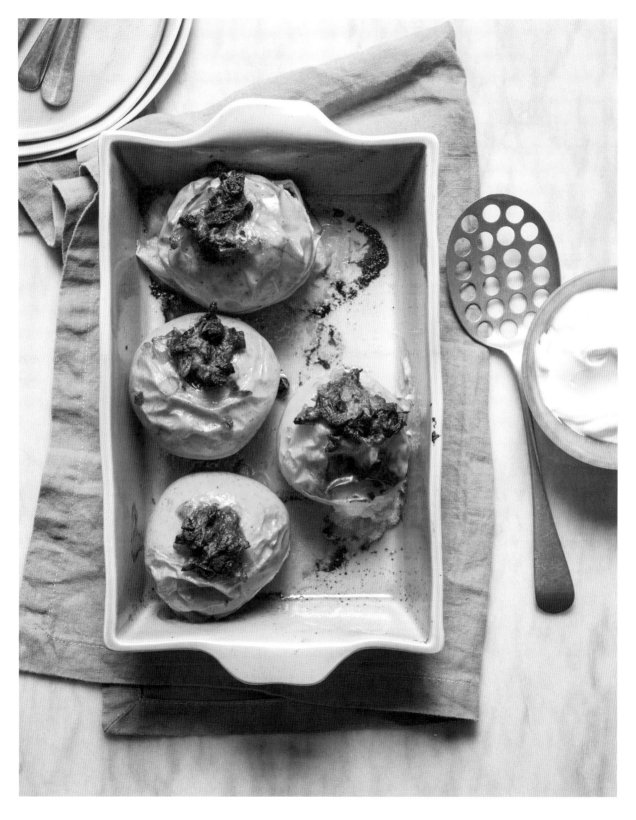

INFO PER APPLE: CALORIES 230   PROTEIN (G) 1.5   CARBS (G) 47   SUGAR (G) 45   FAT (G) 3
SATURATED FAT (G) 1.5   FIBRE (G) 6.5   SALT (G) TRACE

PEANUT BUTTER & OAT COOKIES

75g wholemeal plain flour

25g porridge oats

¼ tsp bicarbonate of soda

pinch of salt

30g golden granulated sugar

50ml maple syrup

125g smooth peanut butter

½ tsp vanilla extract

50g raisins or dark chocolate chips

1–2 tbsp milk

It's not hard to make your own biscuits and that way you know exactly what's in them and can keep track of what you're putting in your body. We've noticed that some people like a soft cookie, while others like more of a crisp biscuit, good for dunking in your cup of tea. With this versatile recipe we've catered for both tastes – if you like a crisper result, just cook the cookies for longer. To make them vegan, use plant-based milk instead of regular.

Preheat the oven to 180°C/Fan 160°C/Gas 4. Line a large baking tray with baking parchment.

Put the flour, oats and bicarbonate of soda in a bowl and add a good pinch of salt.

Put the sugar and maple syrup in a separate large bowl and beat in the peanut butter until the mixture is smooth and aerated. Add the vanilla extract, then all the dry ingredients plus the raisins or chocolate chips. The mixture will probably be quite crumbly at this stage. Add just enough milk to bind the mixture into a smooth, firm dough.

Divide the mixture into 12 small balls. Place them, well-spaced out, on the baking tray, then flatten them down with a fork. Bake for 12 minutes until they're browning around the edges for a soft cookie, or for up to another 5 minutes for a crisper biscuit. They should be fairly flat and have a cracked appearance.

Remove the cookies from the oven and transfer them to a wire rack to cool. Store in an airtight container.

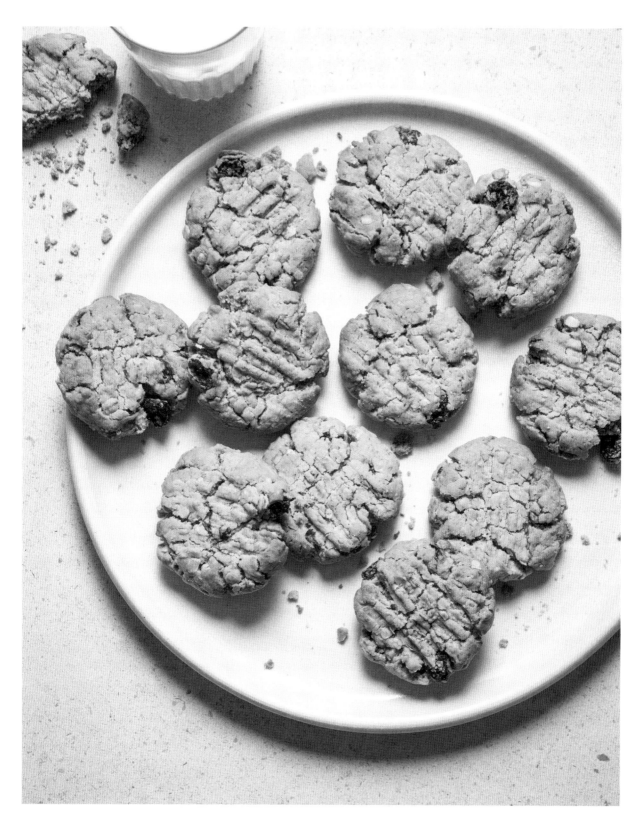

INFO PER COOKIE: CALORIES 129 PROTEIN (G) 3.5 CARBS (G) 14.5 SUGAR (G) 8.5 FAT (G) 6
SATURATED FAT (G) 1.5 FIBRE (G) 1.5 SALT (G) TRACE

MINI MALT LOAVES

vegetable oil, for greasing
175g plain wholemeal flour
2 tsp baking powder
½ tsp bicarbonate of soda
pinch of salt
200g malt extract
75g strong hot tea
50g soft medjool dates, pitted
    weight, finely chopped
100g raisins
1 egg

Glaze
1 tsp malt extract
1 tbsp hot tea

Generations have enjoyed a slice of malt loaf with a cup of tea and with our healthier low-fat version you can carry on the tradition. You don't have to add the glaze but it does give a nice glossy finish and it doesn't take a minute to do. It's worth making these well in advance, as they become stickier and darker after a few days, so be patient and you'll be rewarded. Obviously, you could make one big loaf but these mini loaves are fun and very useful for lunch box portions. You can get special mini loaf tins and we find they come in very useful for all sorts of cakes.

Preheat the oven to 150°C/Fan 130°C/Gas 2. Lightly oil a 12-hole mini loaf tin.

Put the flour, baking powder and bicarb into a bowl and add a generous pinch of salt. Mix thoroughly.

Measure the malt extract into a separate large bowl – the easiest thing is to pour it directly from the jar into the bowl, as it is very sticky and elastic. Pour in the hot tea and stir until the malt extract has dissolved into the tea and you have a texture similar to a thick, pourable syrup. Add the dates and raisins and stir, breaking up any clumps of dates – they will stick together if left to their own devices. Beat in the egg.

Now stir the flour into the bowl to make a mixture with a very loose dropping consistency. Divide the mixture between the individual holes in the tin. Bake in the oven for about 25 minutes until well risen and golden brown. Remove from the oven and leave to cool in the tin. If you do want to make one big loaf in a 900g tin, it will take about an hour to bake.

Mix the malt extract and hot tea together and brush it over the cakes.

Store the cakes in an airtight tin and try to leave them for at least 2 or 3 days before eating. They will be quite light in colour, but will darken and become stickier the longer they are left.

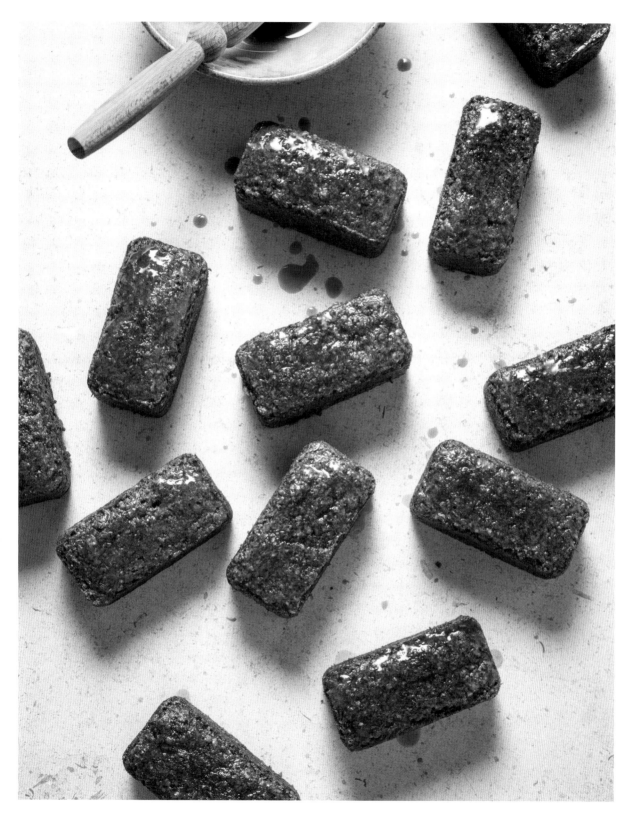

INFO PER MINI LOAF: CALORIES 146 PROTEIN (G) 3.5 CARBS (G)30 SUGAR (G) 20 FAT (G) 1
SATURATED FAT (G) 0   FIBRE (G) 2   SALT (G) TRACE

LEMON & POPPY SEED LOAF CAKE

125g plain live yoghurt

75ml olive oil

100g golden caster sugar or xylitol

3 tbsp honey

3 medium eggs

zest of 2 lemons

125g ground almonds

100g plain flour

2 tsp baking powder

2 tbsp poppy seeds

pinch of salt

A lovely traditional loaf cake, this is made with yoghurt and oil instead of butter and tastes like a dream. If you like, you can use the sweetener xylitol instead of sugar and the flavour is still great. .

Preheat the oven to 180°C/Fan 160°C/Gas 4 and line a 900g loaf tin with baking parchment.

Put the yoghurt, oil, sugar or xylitol, honey, eggs and lemon zest into a large mixing bowl. Whisk until everything is thoroughly combined.

In a separate bowl, mix the ground almonds, flour, baking powder and poppy seeds with a generous pinch of salt. Fold the dry ingredients gently into the wet to form a smooth batter, keeping the mixing to a minimum.

Pour the batter into the prepared loaf tin then bake in the preheated oven for 35–40 minutes until well risen and golden brown. Leave for 5 minutes before removing the cake from the tin.

Serve warm or cold on its own or with yoghurt or crème fraiche.

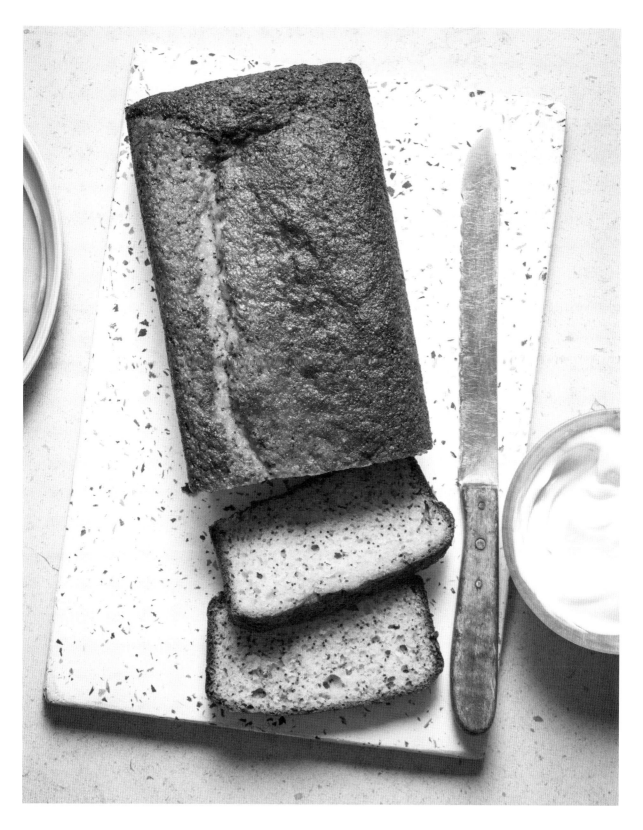

INFO PER SLICE WITH SUGAR/WITH XYLITOL: CALORIES 342/320   PROTEIN (G) 9/9   CARBS (G) 30/25
SUGAR (G) 20/14.5   FAT (G) 20/20   SATURATED FAT (G) 3/3   FIBRE (G) 0.5/0.5   SALT (G) 0.6/0.6

SIDES

& BASICS

WHITE BEAN MASH

INFO PER SERVING: CALORIES 249   PROTEIN (G) 14   CARBS (G) 31   SUGAR (G) 1.5   FAT (G) 4.5   SATURATED FAT (G) 1   FIBRE (G) 13   SALT (G) TRACE

75ml milk

4 garlic cloves

3 x 400g cans of cannellini or butter beans (drained weight is about 750g)

1 tbsp olive oil

small bunch of parsley, finely chopped (or herbs of your choice)

sea salt and black pepper

This is a nice alternative to potato mash. It's just as good for soaking up gravy and juices, but it's higher in fibre and counts towards your five a day. We like to add plenty of herbs – whatever goes well with your main dish.

Pour the milk into a saucepan. Peel the garlic cloves and very thinly slice 3 of them. Add them to the milk and bring up to just below boiling point, then leave to simmer gently until the garlic is tender. This will take about 5 minutes.

Finely grate or crush the remaining garlic clove and add it to the pan with the beans and a generous amount of salt and pepper. Heat until piping hot, then mash or purée. Beat in the olive oil and the parsley or other herbs.

Serves: **4**   Prep: **10 minutes**   Cooking time: **about 25 minutes**

CELERIAC MASH

INFO PER SERVING: CALORIES 116   PROTEIN (G) 3.5   CARBS (G) 15.5   SUGAR (G) 3.5   FAT (G) 2.5
SATURATED FAT (G) 1   FIBRE (G) 10   SALT (G) TRACE

250g floury potatoes, diced
1 celeriac, peeled and diced
    (about 500g unpeeled)
1 tbsp crème fraiche
sea salt and black pepper

You can make a tasty mash with just celeriac, but we like to add some potato to the mix for a bit of extra oomph and texture. About two thirds celeriac to one third potato works well.

Put the potatoes and celeriac in a steamer basket. Season with salt and set the steamer over a pan of boiling water. Cover and steam for 15–20 minutes until tender.

Remove the steamer from the pan, take off the lid and cover with a tea towel for 5 minutes – this will help dry out the vegetables.

Mash, or push the veg through a ricer, then season again with salt and pepper. Beat in the crème fraiche and serve at once.

TOMATO & RED ONION SALAD

INFO PER SERVING: CALORIES 43   PROTEIN (G) 1   CARBS (G) 5.5   SUGAR (G) 4.5   FAT (G) 1.5   SATURATED FAT (G) 0   FIBRE (G) 1.5   SALT (G) TRACE

1 small red onion, finely sliced
   into crescents
300g mixed tomatoes, sliced
   or chopped
1 tbsp capers, rinsed
leaves from a fresh oregano sprig
leaves from a few parsley sprigs,
   finely chopped
sea salt and black pepper

Dressing
2 tsp olive oil
1 tsp sherry vinegar
zest of ½ lemon
¼ tsp sweet or hot paprika
pinch of sugar

We like this simple tomato salad with the cod and ham croquettes on page 68. Just be sure to serve it at room temperature – fridge-cold tomatoes are disappointing and don't taste of anything.

First put the red onion in a bowl, sprinkle it with salt and cover with water. Leave to stand for half an hour, then drain. Mix with the tomatoes, capers and herbs, then season with a little salt and plenty of pepper.

Whisk the dressing ingredients together with pinches of sugar and salt, then add a grinding of pepper. Pour the dressing over the salad and serve at room temperature.

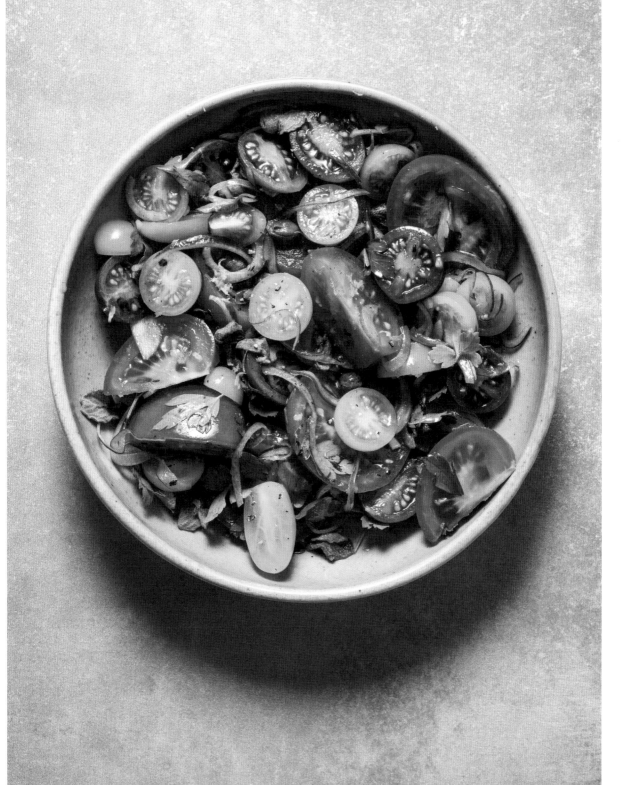

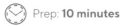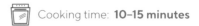

CAULIFLOWER PILAF

INFO PER SERVING: CALORIES 116   PROTEIN (G) 5   CARBS (G) 12   SUGAR (G) 9   FAT (G) 5   SATURATED FAT (G) O.5   FIBRE (G) 3   SALT (G) TRACE

500g cauliflower florets
1 tsp olive oil
1 small onion, finely chopped
25g raisins
½ tsp ground turmeric
¼ tsp ground cinnamon
¼ tsp ground cardamom
sea salt and black pepper

To garnish
25g toasted almonds
leaves from a few mint sprigs
leaves from a few parsley sprigs

A doddle to prepare, this is a great low-cal alternative to a rice pilaf. It goes really well with the Moroccan chicken recipe on page 74.

Put the cauliflower florets in a food processor and pulse to the texture of fine breadcrumbs.

Heat the olive oil in a sauté pan and add the onion and a splash of water. Sauté over a medium heat until softened and lightly golden, then add the raisins and spices. Stir to combine, then add the cauliflower, 50ml of water and plenty of salt and pepper.

Cook the cauliflower for about 5 minutes, stirring regularly, until the mixture looks quite dry and the cauliflower is no longer matt in appearance.

Tip into a serving dish and garnish with the almonds and herbs.

RICE & PEAS

INFO PER SERVING: CALORIES 265   PROTEIN (G) 9.5   CARBS (G) 52.5   SUGAR (G) 1   FAT (G) O
SATURATED FAT (G) O   FIBRE (G) 3.5   SALT (G) TRACE

200g long-grain rice, well rinsed
2 garlic cloves, finely chopped
¼ tsp ground allspice
400ml vegetable stock or water
1 large thyme sprig
1 scotch bonnet, left whole and
    pierced with a knife (optional)
100g cooked brown lentils
2 spring onions, finely sliced
    (whites and greens)
sea salt and black pepper

Traditionally, you would use gungo peas or pigeon peas for this or red kidney beans, but we like this brown lentil version. It's just right with the spiced fish on page 106.

Put the rice in a lidded saucepan with the garlic. Sprinkle over the allspice and season with salt and pepper. Pour in the stock or water, add the thyme and the scotch bonnet, if using, then bring to the boil. Cover and turn down the heat to a simmer. Cook for about 20 minutes or until all the water is absorbed and the rice is tender.

Add the lentils and spring onions to the rice and gently stir them in. Put a tea towel over the saucepan and replace the lid. Leave to stand off the heat for 10 minutes to absorb any excess moisture and ensure the rice is fluffy.

Fish out the thyme sprig and scotch bonnet before serving.

Serves: **4**   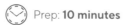 Prep: **10 minutes**   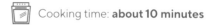 Cooking time: **about 10 minutes**

ASPARAGUS SALAD

INFO PER SERVING: CALORIES 59   PROTEIN (G) 3   CARBS (G) 3   SUGAR (G) 2.5   FAT (G) 3.5
SATURATED FAT (G) 0.5   FIBRE (G) 2.5   SALT (G) TRACE

2 bunches of asparagus
a few mint leaves, finely chopped
a few parsley leaves, finely
   chopped

Dressing
1 tbsp olive oil
1 tbsp lemon juice
1 tsp sherry vinegar
1 tsp pomegranate molasses,
   plus extra if needed
a pinch of chilli flakes
1 preserved lemon, skin only,
   finely chopped
sea salt and black pepper

This is a lovely fresh, simple salad or side dish. We've been sparing with the dressing and kept it quite tart, which we think works well with the asparagus, but feel free to add a little more molasses if your taste buds demand it.

Bend each asparagus spear until it snaps and discard the woody end. Wash the spears thoroughly and shake to get rid of any excess water.

Heat a griddle pan until it's too hot to hold your hand over. Arrange the asparagus spears on the griddle and cook for several minutes, turning regularly until they're all covered in char lines and tender to the point of a knife.

Whisk all the dressing ingredients together and season with salt and pepper. Taste and add a little more pomegranate molasses if you feel it needs it. Drizzle the dressing over the asparagus, then sprinkle with the herbs and serve.

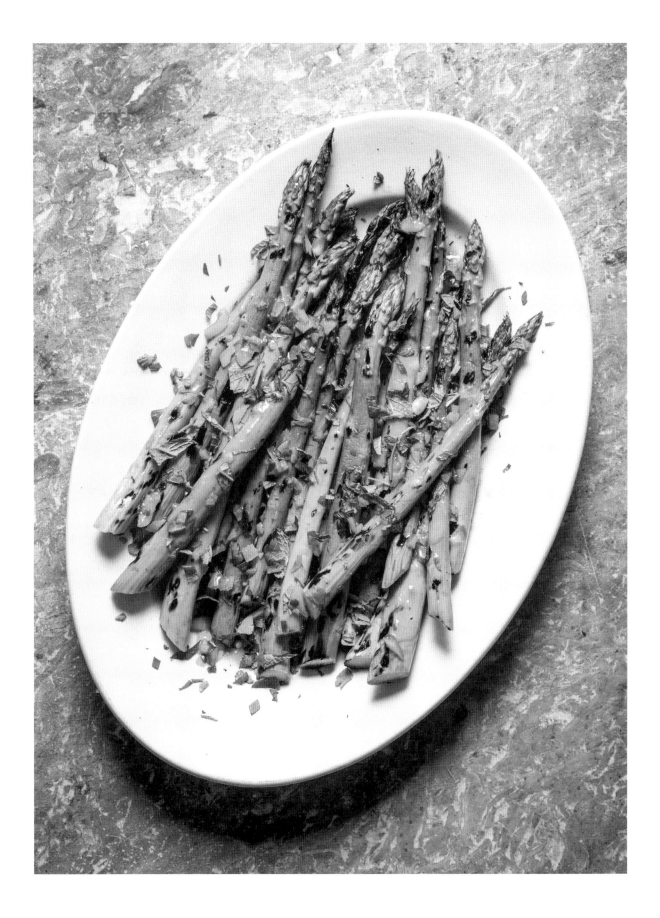

KIMCHI

INFO PER 100G: CALORIES 38   PROTEIN (G) 2   CARBS (G) 3.5   SUGAR (G) 3.5   FAT (G) 1   SATURATED FAT (G) 0   FIBRE (G) 3   SALT (G) 2.7

400g kale or 200g kale and 200g cabbage

1 large carrot, grated or cut into matchsticks

1 large leek, finely sliced into rounds

100g radishes, finely sliced

20g sea salt

spring or filtered water

Paste

1–3 tsp chilli powder, to taste

1 tbsp sweet paprika

1 tsp honey

10g root ginger, grated

2 garlic cloves, crushed

1 small piece of fresh turmeric root, grated or 1 tsp ground turmeric

1 tsp mustard seeds

2 tbsp fish sauce or soy sauce

A Korean staple food, kimchi, or fermented vegetables has become hugely popular recently, as it is reckoned to be really good for your gut. You can buy it ready made in supermarkets, but it's even better if you make it yourself. We did include a recipe in our book 'Everyday Winners', and this is a variation.

First prepare a 1-litre jar. To sterilise it, put it through a hot dishwasher cycle or wash it in hot, soapy water, then rinse thoroughly and leave to dry in a low oven. Make sure the jar is completely dry before filling.

Shred the kale across the stem or remove the stems and keep the leaves in long strips. If using cabbage as well, shred it finely. Put the kale or kale and cabbage in a bowl with the carrot, leek and radishes. Sprinkle over the salt and rub it into the vegetables until they start to release liquid – it will start with a few droplets of water appearing on the surface. Cover with a plate and weigh it down with tins. Leave the vegetables to stand for at least 2 hours, then drain – quite a bit of liquid will have come out of them. Rinse the vegetables with the spring or filtered water, then taste for saltiness. If it's still too salty, rinse again and drain thoroughly.

Mix all the paste ingredients together and pour over the vegetables. Stir to combine, then pack everything into your prepared jar, pushing it all down to make sure there are no air pockets. Seal and leave somewhere cool and dark for 24 hours.

Remove the lid and press everything down again, then reseal and leave for another 24 hours. You should start to see small bubbles appear on the surface and the kimchi should smell pleasantly sour. At this point, you can put the jar in the fridge or leave it fermenting at room temperature for up to 2 weeks, tasting daily until it has the flavour you like. Once you put it in the fridge it will keep fermenting and improving in flavour, but the process will slow down considerably. The kimchi will keep in the fridge indefinitely.

Makes: **500g fairly strong-tasting, thick kefir**   Prep: **15 minutes + fermenting**

KEFIR

INFO PER 100G: CALORIES 63   PROTEIN (G) 3.4   CARBS (G) 4.5   SUGAR (G) 4.5   FAT (G) 3.5
SATURATED FAT (G) 2.5   FIBRE (G) 0   SALT (G) TRACE

10g activated kefir grains
500ml whole milk, preferably
    organic, even better, raw organic

Our mate Chris Thompson swears by kefir for keeping him and his family in tip-top condition, so we're giving it a go. There are lots of different versions, but this is a good one for starters. You have to begin by activating the kefir grains, so just follow the instructions provided with them.

Prepare your equipment. You will need a large glass jar – a Kilner one is ideal. You don't need to sterilise it, but do wash it in very hot soapy water and dry it thoroughly.

Put the activated kefir grains in the prepared jar and add the milk. Make sure the jar allows for several centimetres of headroom at the top. If using a Kilner jar of the sort that has a rubber seal, close the lid without the seal. Otherwise, cover the jar with a double layer of muslin or cheesecloth, or a couple of pieces of kitchen paper. Secure this with string or rubber bands.

Leave the jar at room temperature (18°C or above – the warmer it is, the shorter the ferment time) and out of direct sunlight for 18–24 hours. Stir every 6 hours, if you remember. It should thicken in that time, but if it doesn't it will probably be because the temperature has dipped. If it is a very hot day, the kefir might ferment in just a few hours. When it has thickened, taste and leave it for longer if you want a stronger flavour.

Strain the kefir through a sieve to retrieve the grains. You can start the process again with some or all of the grains (they do grow over time). If you don't want to use them immediately, cover the grains with milk and leave them in the fridge until needed. You can also freeze grains for up to 6 months, then reactivate them.

Store the kefir in the fridge. It will continue to ferment very gently and should be edible for up to a month.

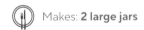 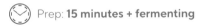

RAINBOW SAUERKRAUT

INFO PER 100G: CALORIES 31   PROTEIN (G) 1   CARBS (G) 4.5   SUGAR (G) 4   FAT (G) 0
SATURATED FAT (G) 0   FIBRE (G) 3   SALT (G) 1.6

½ red cabbage, about 250g

½ white or green pointed cabbage, about 250g

400g mixed vegetables – carrots, red pepper, beetroots, rainbow chard, kale, leek, celeriac, radishes, turnips, garlic

a few sprigs of herbs (parsley, mint, coriander, thyme, dill), finely chopped

1 tbsp sea salt

1 tsp mustard seeds

1 tbsp grated fresh turmeric root or 1 tsp ground

spring or filter water

This is wonderful stuff to have in the fridge and makes a delicious side dish or snack. Just follow the method carefully and you can't go wrong.

Wash 2 large wide-rimmed preserving jars and dry them thoroughly.

Shred the cabbages and all the other vegetables as finely as you can. Root vegetables can be grated or cut into matchstick strips. Put them all in a large bowl. Add the herbs, but be sparing, as they will carry a lot of flavour. Add the sea salt and rub it into the vegetables until they start to give out liquid – droplets will start to appear on the surface – and you'll feel the texture change. Keep massaging until the cabbage looks wet and is sitting in a pool of water. If it's resistant, you can weigh it down and leave it to stand for an hour.

Stir in the mustard seeds and turmeric, then pack the vegetables into the jars, pressing them down as much as possible to make sure there are no air bubbles. You'll need enough room at the top of each jar to weigh the veg down, so don't fill them more than three-quarters full.

Divide any liquid left in the bowl between the jars. If it doesn't quite cover the vegetables, add a small amount of filtered or spring water. Weigh down the vegetables with special glass weights or use plastic bags filled with water. Or if there's room, you can use a couple of shallow ramekins. Make sure that all the vegetables are sitting below the surface of the liquid, as it's important that they don't come into contact with the air. Seal the jars.

Leave them somewhere cool and dark for several days, checking every day and loosening the lid every day to make sure the build up of gases within the jars is released. You should start to see small air bubbles appear after 24 hours. Taste the sauerkraut after 4 or 5 days. If you are happy with what should be a pleasantly sour flavour, remove the weights and transfer the jars to the fridge. The sauerkraut will keep fermenting at a much slower rate. Start eating it immediately or leave it for up to several months. Once opened, eat within a few weeks.

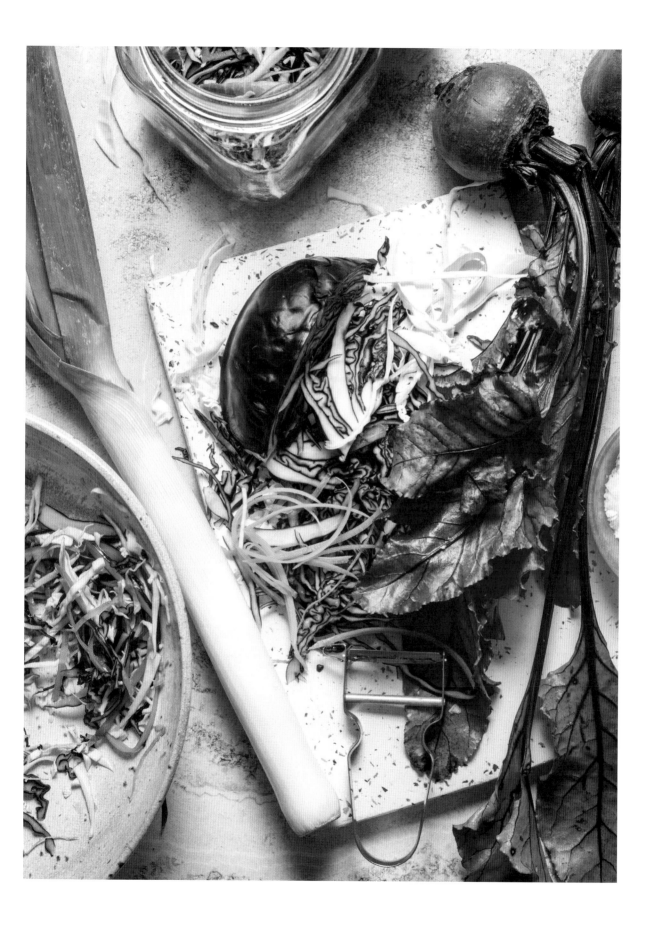

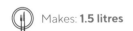
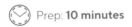
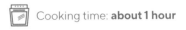
VEGETABLE STOCK

1 tsp olive oil
2 large onions, roughly chopped
3 large carrots, chopped
200g squash or pumpkin,
   unpeeled, diced
4 celery sticks, sliced
2 leeks, sliced
100ml white wine or vermouth
a large thyme sprig
a large parsley sprig
1 bay leaf
a few peppercorns

Stock is a great way of using up any slightly past their best vegetables at the bottom of the fridge – and it will make your soups taste even better.

Heat the olive oil in a large saucepan. Add all the vegetables and fry them over a high heat, stirring regularly, until they start to brown and caramelise around the edges. This will take at least 10 minutes. Add the white wine or vermouth and boil until it has evaporated away.

Cover the vegetables with 2 litres of water and add the herbs and peppercorns. Bring to the boil, then turn the heat down to a gentle simmer. Cook the stock, uncovered, for about an hour, stirring every so often.

Check the stock – the colour should have some depth to it. Strain it through a colander or a sieve lined with muslin or kitchen paper into a bowl. Store it in the fridge for up to a week or freeze it.

FISH STOCK

1.5kg fish heads and bones from white fish
1 tbsp salt
2 tbsp olive oil
1 onion, finely chopped
2 leeks, finely sliced
½ fennel bulb, finely chopped
1 celery stick, sliced
2 garlic cloves, sliced
200ml white wine
bouquet garni made up of 2 sprigs each of parsley, tarragon and thyme
2 bay leaves
a few peppercorns
1 piece of thinly pared lemon zest

Your fishmonger will give you fish heads and bones for stock. White fish, such as cod, haddock and sole, are best, but avoid oily fish.

Put the fish heads and bones in a bowl, cover them with cold water and add the salt. Leave to stand for an hour, then drain and wash thoroughly under running water. This process helps to draw out any blood from the fish and gives you a clearer, fresher-tasting stock.

Heat the olive oil in a large saucepan. Add the onion, leeks, fennel, celery and garlic. Cook the vegetables over a medium heat for several minutes until they start to soften without taking on any colour.

Add the fish heads and bones and pour over the wine. Bring to the boil, then add 2 litres of water. Bring back to the boil, skim off any mushroom-coloured foam that appears on the surface, then turn the heat down to a very slow simmer. Add the herbs, peppercorns and lemon zest and leave to simmer for 30 minutes, skimming off any foam every so often.

Strain the stock through a colander or sieve into a bowl, then line the sieve with muslin or kitchen paper and strain the stock again. Don't push it through as that will result in a cloudier stock. Leave to cool, then keep in the fridge for 3–4 days or freeze it.

CHICKEN STOCK

at least 1 chicken carcass,
   pulled apart

4 chicken wings (optional)

1 onion, unpeeled, cut into
   quarters

1 large carrot, cut into large chunks

2 celery sticks, roughly chopped

1 leek, roughly chopped

1 tsp black peppercorns

3 bay leaves

a large parsley sprig

a small thyme sprig

a few garlic cloves, unpeeled
   (optional)

Once you've enjoyed your Sunday roast, don't throw the chicken carcass away. Use it to make a delicious stock to enrich your dishes. You can also buy chicken carcasses very cheaply at most butchers.

Put the chicken bones and the wings, if using, into a saucepan, just large enough for all the chicken to fit quite snugly. Cover with cold water, bring to the boil, then skim off any foam that collects. Add the remaining ingredients and turn the heat down to a very low simmer. Partially cover the pan with a lid.

Leave the stock to simmer for about 3 hours, then remove the pan from the heat. Strain the stock through a colander or a sieve lined with muslin or kitchen paper into a bowl.

The stock can be used right away, although it is best to skim off most of the fat that will collect on the top. If you don't need the stock immediately, leave it to cool. The fat will set on top and will be much easier to remove.

You can keep the stock in the fridge for up to 5 days or freeze it. If you want to make a larger amount of stock, save up your chicken carcasses in the freezer or add more chicken wings.

BEEF STOCK

1.5.kg beef bones, including
marrow bones, if possible,
cut into small lengths
500g piece of beef shin or any
cheap, fairly lean cut
2 onions, unpeeled, roughly
chopped
1 leek, roughly chopped
2 celery sticks, roughly chopped
2 carrots, roughly chopped
2 tomatoes
½ tsp peppercorns
bouquet garni made up of large
sprigs of thyme, parsley and
2 bay leaves

Proper beef stock does need to simmer for quite a long time but it's no trouble to make and adds loads of flavour to stews and casseroles.

Put the beef bones and meat into a large saucepan and cover them with cold water – at least 3–3.5 litres. Bring the water to the boil and when a starchy, mushroom-grey foam appears, start skimming. Keep on skimming as the foam turns white and continue until it has almost stopped developing.

Add the vegetables, peppercorns and bouquet garni, turn down the heat until the stock is simmering very gently, then partially cover the pan with a lid. Leave to simmer for 3–4 hours.

Line a sieve or colander with 2 layers of muslin or a clean tea towel and place it over a large bowl. Ladle the stock into the sieve or colander to strain it. Remove the meat and set it aside, then discard everything else. Pour the strained stock into a large container and leave it to cool. The fat should solidify on top of the stock and will be very easy to remove. You can keep the stock in the fridge for 2 or 3 days or freeze it.

Don't chuck out the piece of meat – it's good in sandwiches or it can be sliced, fried and added to salads.

INDEX

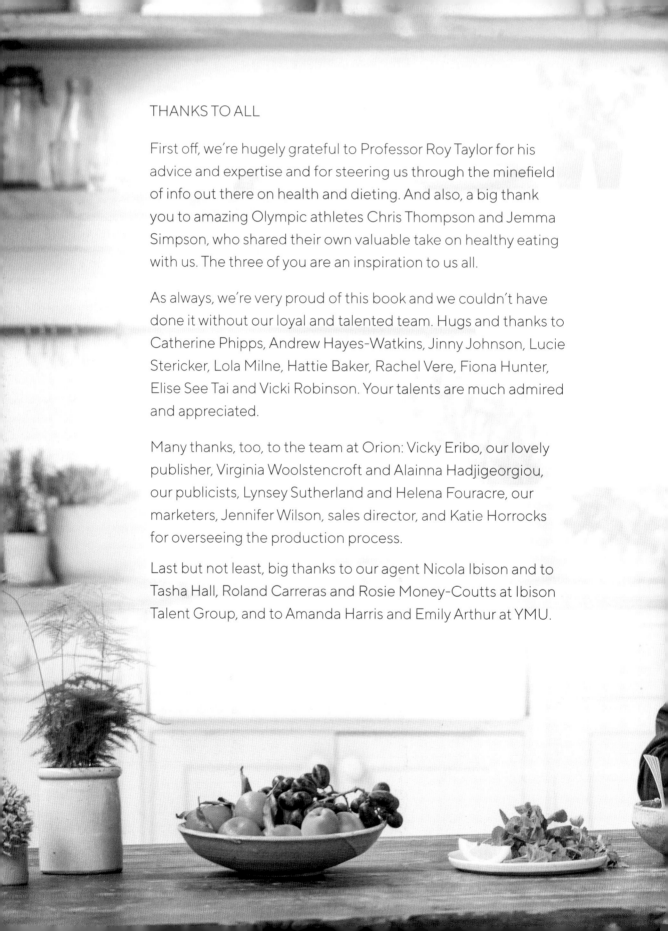

THANKS TO ALL

First off, we're hugely grateful to Professor Roy Taylor for his advice and expertise and for steering us through the minefield of info out there on health and dieting. And also, a big thank you to amazing Olympic athletes Chris Thompson and Jemma Simpson, who shared their own valuable take on healthy eating with us. The three of you are an inspiration to us all.

As always, we're very proud of this book and we couldn't have done it without our loyal and talented team. Hugs and thanks to Catherine Phipps, Andrew Hayes-Watkins, Jinny Johnson, Lucie Stericker, Lola Milne, Hattie Baker, Rachel Vere, Fiona Hunter, Elise See Tai and Vicki Robinson. Your talents are much admired and appreciated.

Many thanks, too, to the team at Orion: Vicky Eribo, our lovely publisher, Virginia Woolstencroft and Alainna Hadjigeorgiou, our publicists, Lynsey Sutherland and Helena Fouracre, our marketers, Jennifer Wilson, sales director, and Katie Horrocks for overseeing the production process.

Last but not least, big thanks to our agent Nicola Ibison and to Tasha Hall, Roland Carreras and Rosie Money-Coutts at Ibison Talent Group, and to Amanda Harris and Emily Arthur at YMU.

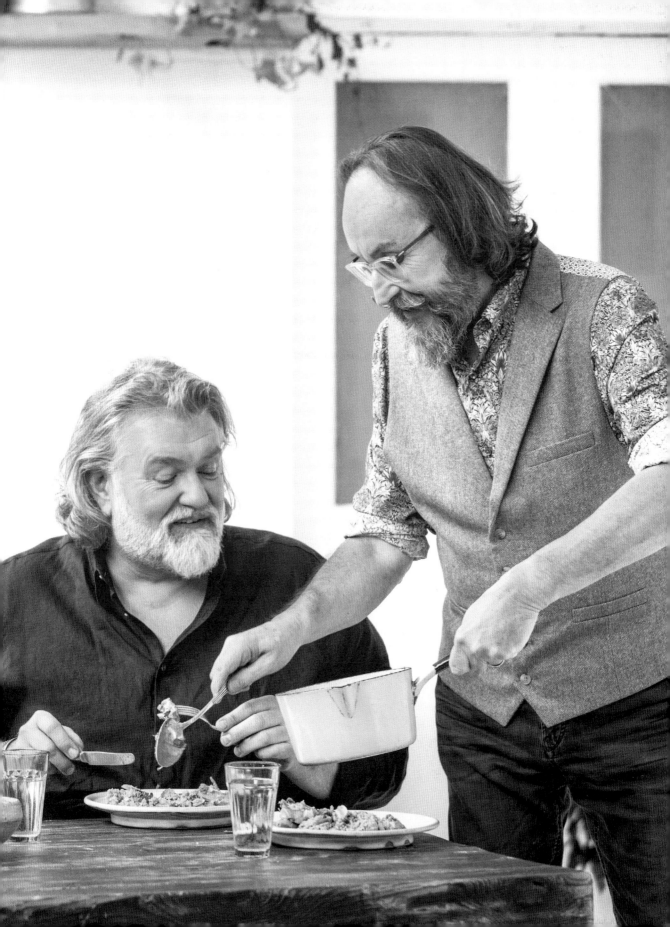

We'd like to dedicate this book to Roy Taylor, whose advice ten years ago when we started our Healthy Dieters series has stood us in very good stead. Roy has been tough yet supportive and always good humoured – for this, we thank you.

First published in Great Britain in 2022 by Seven Dials,
an imprint of The Orion Publishing Group Ltd
Carmelite House, 50 Victoria Embankment
London EC4Y 0DZ

An Hachette UK Company

13 5 7 9 10 8 6 4 2

ISBN (Hardback) 978 1 8418 8433 2
ISBN (eBook) 978 1 8418 8434 9

Publisher: Vicky Eribo
Recipe consultant: Catherine Phipps
Photography: Andrew Hayes-Watkins
Design and art direction: Lucie Stericker, Studio 7:15
Editor: Jinny Johnson
Food stylist: Lola Milne
Food stylist's assistant: Hattie Baker

Prop stylist: Rachel Vere
Proofreader: Elise See Tai
Indexer: Vicki Robinson
Production manager: Katie Horrocks

Nutritional information calculated by Fiona Hunter,
    Bsc (Hons) Nutrition, Dip Dietetics

Printed in Germany

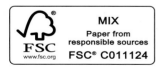

www.orionbooks.co.uk